"Only in recent years has the importance of core strength, which involves the muscles of the abdomen, the back, and the pelvis, been fully recognized. The author has addressed this subject in a very scientific yet practical way. She describes how one can analyze their personal need for fitness and then how to improve their fitness level by doing simple core exercises, which progressively become more difficult. The exercises are well illustrated and easily understood. I can highly recommend this book for anyone who has the desire to improve their fitness level and their lifestyle."

—Robert W. Jackson, OC, MD, FRCS(C), chief emeritus in the Department of Orthopaedic Surgery at Baylor University Medical Center

"As a former Olympic athlete in alpine skiing, and now working professional, I had suffered and continue to suffer from periodic back ailments, and I would definitely tell my friends that *Solid to the Core* is a must read."

—Jim Kirby, former Olympian, member of the Canadian National Ski Team, and general manager of the sports section at Publicis Canada

"*Solid to the Core* is a great resource book for all athletes and rehabilitation specialists. The exercises and progressions allow all athletes to continually challenge their core musculature. This can only enhance your overall athletic performance and health."

—Chris Broadhurst, CAI(c), head athletic therapist for the Phoenix Coyotes Hockey Team

"Anything written by Janique Farand-Taylor is worth reading. It could change your life. Working out with Janique as my instructor for the past five years has certainly changed mine—for the better. She makes a difference."

—Ted Rogers, president and CEO of Rogers Communications, Inc., in Toronto, ON, Canada

"It used to be that 'training' meant going into the gym and doing a few bench presses. But no more. Now everyone involved in athletics recognizes the need for building a strong stable foundation for the body. Core training is important to everyone from fitness exercisers to professional athletes, and Janique knows core training. This is a great program—and it works."

—Nick Kypreos, analyst with Rogers Sportsnet and 1994 Stanley Cup champion with the New York Rangers

solid
to the core

SIMPLE EXERCISES TO INCREASE
CORE STRENGTH & FLEXIBILITY

JANIQUE FARAND-TAYLOR, PT, ACE
FOREWORD BY IAN FINKELSTEIN, MD

New Harbinger Publications, Inc.

Distributed in Canada by Raincoast Books.

Copyright © 2006 by Janique Farand-Taylor
New Harbinger Publications, Inc.
5674 Shattuck Avenue
Oakland, CA 94609
www.newharbinger.com

Cover design by Amy Shoup
Cover and interior photography by Jean Desjardins
Text design by Michele Waters-Kermes
Acquired by Melissa Kirk
Edited by Brady Kahn

Printed in the United States of America

Library of Congress Cataloging-in-Publication Data

Farand-Taylor, Janique.
   Solid to the core : simple exercises to increase core strength and flexibility / Janique Farand-Taylor.
        p. cm.
   ISBN 1-57224-430-5
   1. Exercise. 2. Physical fitness. 3. Exercise therapy. I. Title.
   RA781.F35 2006
   613.7'1—dc22
                                         2005037403

08   07   06

10   9   8   7   6   5   4   3   2   1

First printing

To Jessica, Chloé, and Danika, who are my inspiration in life. To Alexantoine and Guillaume, who made me pursue my passion. To Anabel, Christophe, and Claudie-Anne, who are far away but always in my mind.

Contents

Foreword

Chronic musculoskeletal pain is a major health problem affecting nearly one third of the population, accounts for almost 50% of chronic pain complaints and is responsible for approximately 20% of visits to a primary care physician. It carries large direct and indirect health care costs, with most available financial data focusing on back pain. It has been associated with deficits in quality of life and psychological adjustment, disability, reduced income potential, high levels of health care utilization and high costs to private industry. Regardless of its underlying cause, gaining control over chronic musculoskeletal pain can pose a treatment challenge to clinicians and therapists alike.

Unfortunately, much of how we deliver health care today is still based on the treatment of disease and illness rather than placing emphasis on prevention. Improved level of fitness, proper diet and maintaining a health bodyweight will all go far to prevent the onset of disease or potential for injury. Developing a strong and stable core musculature around the spine along with proper postural alignment, will allow for improved balance, flexibility and endurance.

Muscle imbalance or postural abnormalities can cause or influence numerous orthopedic and neurologic diseases and syndromes of pain and impairment. Often we see patients at our clinic who have been suffering from chronic pain secondary to musculoskeletal imbalance. We have developed an active rehabilitation program to treat these patients which incorporates the foundations of Janique Farand-Taylor's book. We combine this program with Botox® injections into the overactive and tight muscles. This integrative approach aims to restore muscle imbalance, reduce pain and improve the patient's overall posture.

Janique Farand-Taylor provides an innovative and practical program aimed at improving core muscle strength, muscle imbalance and posture in the lumbar/pelvic area. She skillfully blends simplicity of use and time efficiency into a comprehensive and progressive program that will appeal to everyone. Whether you are healthy, injured or are in chronic pain, this book will provide a strong foundation by which you can improve your overall level of strength, endurance and function. I applaud her work, recommend it as a must read to patients, clinicians and therapists alike, and I anxiously await the release of her next book focusing on the neck and shoulder areas.

—Ian Finkelstein, MD, DAAPM
Medical Director of the Toronto Headache and Pain Clinic

Acknowledgments

I would like to express my heartfelt appreciation to the people who have helped me make this book possible.

I want to thank my family, beginning with my husband, Douglas. He provided invaluable assistance looking after our children when I was in dire need of time to write this book. Also, thank you so much to my three beautiful girls, Jessica, Chloé, and Danika, who are my life!

I must also thank my father Gilles, my mother Lucie, and my two sisters, Chantal and Andrée-Anne, who have been an integral influence in every aspect of my life. They spent hours of their precious time participating in all of my activities and decision-making. Thank you for your unconditional love, support, encouragement, advice, and guidance. You taught me so much.

There are various other individuals to whom I am very grateful for their support. I want to thank all of the patients who trusted me with their health and believed in my work. As a sports physiotherapist, it is very rewarding when you can make a difference in someone's life. I must also thank David J. MacLeod, who designed and produced my first lumbo-pelvic stabilization booklet, and Kevin Brown, Monica Piccininno, and Annette Carlucci, of MediaEdge Communications, who skillfully organized, designed, and printed the first edition of *Solid to the Core*. The photographs of the exercises were taken by my friend Jean Desjardins. Thank you, Jean.

My most profound appreciation goes to my agent, Arnold Gosewich, and to New Harbinger Publications for their unlimited devotion. Without their support and assistance, creating the second edition of *Solid to the Core* would have been far more difficult. I owe them my deepest gratitude.

I would also like to recognize Signy Franklin's invaluable contribution to the development of *Solid to the Core*. She not only shared my vision, but also provided useful suggestions and substantive comments about the chapter Swiss Ball Stabilization. Signy also recognized the potential of my ideas and spent long hours putting them on the computer so eloquently. Without her commitment, none of this work would have been completed. Many thanks to Signy for going the extra mile. I greatly appreciate it. She is also the model for the photographs in *Solid to the Core*.

Introduction

This book came about because of the many problems my clients were experiencing with their back, neck, lower, and/or upper extremities. Not having any protocol of exercises that could be adapted to each client, I decided to research the area that was the most problematic: "the core."

Being a sports physiotherapist for more then fifteen years and having encountered a variety of injuries with different patients, I discovered that I could successfully treat injuries, using manual therapeutic techniques, such as soft tissue releases, joints mobilization, craniosacral therapy, and acupuncture. However, if the cause of the original problem was not addressed first, I found that injuries would be more likely to reoccur. This cause—and the root of most patients' discomfort—was an imbalance of the muscles around the core. The core is a group of muscles extending from the base of the spine to the pelvis area. It includes muscles of the abdominal wall, the back, and the pelvis. As I began to realize that this core weakness was a common problem with my clients, I became frustrated when I could find no book that addressed this issue.

The core of our body is similar to the foundation of a house. If the foundation of the house (its core) is not strong, the walls around it (the arms and legs) will be unstable. You can build a beautiful house but without a solid base, the walls will start to fall apart. Similarly, if your arms and legs do not have a stable base of support, then you will suffer from muscle imbalances as you go about your daily activities, such as walking, carrying groceries, or doing household tasks. This is a clear cause-and-effect scenario. The stronger the foundation of your house, the more solid the walls are going to be. For the body to perform well, you must have full control of the spine and the pelvis to prevent any injuries. Core strength is the foundation needed to prevent injuries. In the case of injury, core strengthening exercises are crucial to regaining strength, flexibility, and stability. They also should be the basis of everyone's fitness program. Unfortunately, most people think of core training as "having great abs." But core strength involves much more than having sculpted abdominals. Always remember that it is not only about the aesthetic appeal of a great looking mid-section but also about the functional necessity of a "solid" strong core.

This book's approach is unique in the core strengthening field. While it is based on Joseph Pilates' philosophy that the core muscles are the foundation of all physical movements, it differs in that it takes into consideration muscle imbalances around the core. Rampant poor posture puts the core muscles to sleep, leaving you in a constant belly-bulging slump. You need to retrain and strengthen those belly-slimming, stand-tall muscles to regain good postural alignment.

Developing Good Posture

Good postural alignment means maintaining the natural curves of your spine, as well as keeping your knee, hip, and shoulder joints stacked on top of each other; you should be able to feel the top of your head reaching toward the ceiling, ears over shoulders, chin level at a 90-degree angle, shoulders back, down and relaxed over the hips, hips over knees, knees over ankles, and your weight distributed evenly onto the soles of your feet.

What This Book Will Teach You

This book describes the most effective strength exercises and protocols to train the five most important muscles and muscle groups centered around the spine. These consist of the deep and superficial muscles of the abdominal wall and the lower back as well as the gluteal muscles of the pelvis.

Illustrated here are 84 core strength exercises to help people of all ages. You will learn to customize your core program according to your own weaknesses and muscle imbalances. At first, you will be introduced to some basic concepts and techniques. You will gradually advance to work with the resistance band, medicine ball, and Swiss ball. Photographs reinforce written instructions and ensure proper execution of each technique presented. These exercises were developed from personal experience as well as the experiences of many world-class athletes who experienced injury and weakness due to a weak core, preventing them from pursuing higher training regimens. With this book, you will discover how efficient you can become in your daily activities as you strengthen your body's core.

The Benefits of the Program

You can enjoy all the benefits described below, and more, if you can give twenty minutes a day to performing the core exercise program presented in this book. Helping you move through your hectic life with a strong, flexible, and balanced core is the goal. The key benefits of the Solid to the Core program are as follows:

- to minimize the risk of injuries

- to correct muscle imbalances

- to work for healthy or injured, young or old, sedentary or active, male or female

- to give you better posture and less discomfort

- to make you feel strong, energetic, powerful, and healthy

Ultimately, you will feel so strong, flexible, and balanced that if someone asks you how you feel, your immediate answer will be, "Finally! It's so fantastic! I have no more aches and pains. Thank you, Solid to the Core!

CHAPTER 1

The Basics of Solid to the Core

The muscles of the back are responsible for maintaining posture and allowing the spine to move. But back stabilization is maintained primarily by small, deep muscles that, because of their size and depth, people rarely notice. This exercise program is designed to train the deep muscles of the lower back, the abdominal region, and the pelvis to provide stability to the core of the body. When you train these muscles, the larger and more superficial muscles, which previously compensated for pelvic inadequacies, can relax and become less stressed.

The five core muscles and muscle groups are identifiable by the depth at which they are located. They are the deep flexor abdominal muscle (transversus abdominis), the superficial flexor abdominal muscles (rectus abdominis and obliques), the deep extensor back muscle (multifidus), the superficial extensor back muscle (erector spinae), and the pelvis muscles (gluteals).

Primary Muscle Stabilizers of the Core

The Solid to the Core program focuses on two deep muscles that are the most important for core stabilization: the multifidus muscle and the transversus abdominis. See the first illustration in this chapter (Kapit, Wynn, and Elson 1977).

The *multifidus* is the muscle of strongest influence in the lower back region. It spans five or six vertebrae up the spine. When the body is upright, you need to continuously activate it for support and control. Small movements of the multifidus allow for fine adjustments in the vertebrae of the spine. The muscle of the superficial layer of the back is the *erector spinae* and it runs parallel to the vertebrae of the spine. If the multifidus muscle is dysfunctional and weak, the erector spinae muscle tends to be overworked, resulting in muscle imbalances around the core. Secondary complications, which can be debilitating if you do not correct these imbalances, include upper and lower extremity injuries, such as tendonitis or arthritis.

In the abdominal region, the key stabilization muscle is the *transversus abdominis*. The transversus abdominis starts at the lower spine and attaches horizontally to the ribs, abdominal wall, and pelvis. It supports the abdominal wall by wrapping belt-like around the back and abdomen, creating a decompression of the spine. It also contributes to respiration.

As with the multifidus muscle, properly engaging the transversus abdominis stabilizes the spine and the pelvis, making it possible to use your core as an anchoring system for your upper and lower extremities. To engage your transversus abdominis, draw your abdomen in without holding your breath or forcing your belly button to your spine. Just draw in the entire circumference of your abdomen toward the middle of your lower back. It feels like you are wearing a belt or a girdle.

The proper functioning of the multifidus and the transversus abdominis is the primary goal of this exercise program.

Secondary Muscle Stabilizers of the Core

Your abdominal wall is supported by four muscles. From the most superficial layer to the deepest one, they are the rectus abdominis, the external and internal obliques, and the transversus abdominis (described above).

The *rectus abdominis* is the most superficial and central muscle of the abdominal wall, and it is the one muscle in this area that can be overtrained. Everyone can do curl ups. However, it is easy to overtrain this superficial muscle and ignore the deeper muscles that support the core.

The *external oblique* muscle is the outermost of the three "flat" muscles of the abdominal wall, with the *internal oblique* muscle being the middle and the transversus abdominis muscle the innermost one. The obliques are also very important in the stabilization of the core and are often forgotten.

The *gluteus maximus* is the largest muscle in the whole body. It is a very powerful extensor of the hip and a stabilizer of the hip joint in the erect posture. However, the pelvis is also steadied at each step by the *gluteus medius* muscle, which is an important stabilizer of the pelvis (it tilts the pelvis) in walking and when you are standing on one leg. In these actions, it is assisted by the *gluteus minimus*, which is the smallest of the gluteal muscles. To be able to perform these functions, the gluteal muscles, their levers, and the fulcrum of the movement must be intact. The levers are the *femoral head* and the *femoral neck*, located at the top part of the femoral bone of the thigh; the fulcrum is the hip joint. When any of these structures is not functioning properly, the pelvis will not tilt to the affected side if the opposite foot is raised from the ground. In medical terms, this test is called the "Trendelenburg sign." The gait resulting from a defective Trendelenburg sign will be one in which the affected side dips with each step. It will

Muscular System/The Torso
Deep Muscles of the Back and Neck

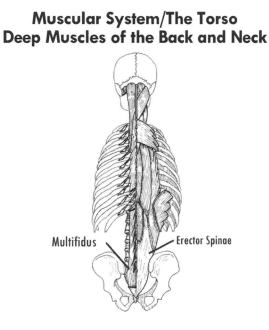

Multifidus   Erector Spinae

Muscular System/The Torso Muscles of the
Anterior Abdominal Wall and Inguinal Region

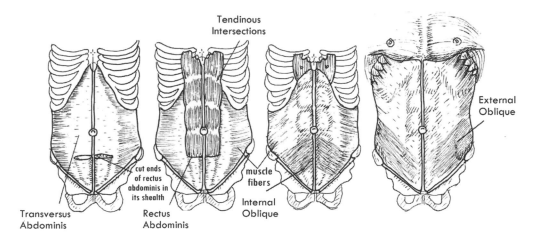

Tendinous
Intersections

External
Oblique

cut ends
of rectus
abdominis in
its sheath

muscle
fibers

Transversus
Abdominis

Rectus
Abdominis

Internal
Oblique

result in muscle imbalances around the core, along with secondary complications, including upper and lower extremity injuries, such as tendonitis or arthritis.

Analyzing Your Fitness Needs

Clearly, no single activity provides full fitness benefits, and everyone has different needs. It's important that you recognize your own fitness needs and injuries early on in the planning and design of your exercise program, because a poor training program design can lead to chronic injuries.

Still, there are some basic elements that are germane to overall fitness: cardiovascular fitness/warm-up, flexibility, and muscular strength. Understanding these as they apply to the Solid to the Core program will better prepare you to analyze the exercises you are about to start doing. If all of these elements are present in your exercise program, you will be more focused on overall fitness.

As you analyze your fitness needs, be sure to consult a physician to make sure you are healthy enough to begin this program.

The Cardiovascular Warm-Up

Cardiovascular training should be part of any exercise regimen because it warms up the muscles. There are four components to cardiovascular fitness: type of activity, how long you do the activity, how strenuous the activity is, and how often the activity is performed. In the fitness world, these four components are called the FITT principle (frequency, intensity, time, and type).

A sound approach to warming up is doing cardiovascular exercises, such as marching, riding a stationary bike, or walking on a treadmill, for five to ten minutes. Most exercisers warm up at low levels of intensity yet develop satisfactory levels of cardiovascular health by increasing the duration and frequency of their workouts over time.

Exercisers often look at their resting heart rate as a measure of their level of cardiovascular fitness. Resting heart rates can vary among individuals, ranging from 45 to 75 beats per minute, from the very fit to those who are less fit, respectively.

To determine your resting heart rate, first find your pulse by pressing your index and long fingers to the side of your wrist or the side of your neck under the jawbone. Count the number of pulses for ten seconds and multiply by six. Do this several times during the day to arrive at a good average for your resting heart rate. You can also use this method to measure your heart rate while exercising.

For greater precision, heart rate monitors are an ideal tool. The most accurate heart rate monitor is a chest strap transmitter, which fits snugly around the chest, just below the bra or the nipples. The chest strap transmitter will detect the activity of your heart and will relay that information to a wristwatch-like receiver. Many people are happy with the basic models that simply display heart rate; more expensive models also offer a zone alarm (it beeps when your heart rate's too high or too low) and calculate calories burned while exercising. You can purchase heart rate monitors at most sporting goods stores.

Your aerobic warm-up should be intense enough to increase your heart rate to 50 to 60 percent of your maximum heart rate. The formula for calculating your maximum heart rate (Max HR) in beats per minute (bpm) is 220 minus your age (in years).

To calculate 50 percent and 60 percent of your Max HR, multiply your Max HR by 0.50 and 0.60. This is your target heart rate (THR), or the range within which your heart rate should stay while warming up. As an example, if you are forty years old and your Max HR is 180 bpm, your formula will look like this:

Age: 40
Max HR: 220 - 40 = 180 bpm
Lower THR: 0.50 x 180 = 90 bpm
Upper THR: 0.60 x 180 = 108 bpm

This formula tells you that your heart rate should be between 90 bpm and 108 bpm while you're warming up. If your heart rate is below 90 bpm, increase the intensity of your exercise, and if it is above 108 bpm, reduce it slightly. You should take your heart rate prior to warming up and every five minutes thereafter.

All warm-ups should be of sufficient intensity to elevate your body temperature. Sweating slightly is a good indication that you are ready to move on to the next phase of your workout: flexibility.

Stretching for Better Flexibility

After you have warmed up for five or ten minutes, you should do some pre-exercise stretching to increase muscle flexibility. To evaluate your flexibility, do the three stretches described below and see if your right and left sides feel symmetrical. If not, you may have started to develop a compensatory pattern, which will result in muscle imbalances. If this is the case, write down which side seems dysfunctional (less flexible, more painful, having less range of motion). Be specific about the exact area where you feel discomfort. You can use the blank lines below to record your evaluations.

1. **Hips and front thighs (quadriceps):** Stand with your back to a wall, about two feet away. Drop to your hands and knees. Slide both knees back to where the wall meets the floor and point your toes up so they are flush against the wall. Slowly bring your left leg in front of you, foot flat on the floor and knee bent at a 90-degree angle so that your left armpit is above your left knee. With both hands on your left knee,

move your torso upward striving to bring it parallel with the wall. Hold for thirty seconds, and repeat with the right side.

If you have any hip or knee problems, try the easy version instead: Drop to your hands and knees. Slowly bring your left leg in front of you, so your foot is flat on the floor and your knee is bent at a 90-degree angle. Bring right leg back with knee touching the floor. Slowly push pelvis forward until a stretch is felt on the front of the right hip.

Evaluation: _____

(Example: "Right front thigh, middle area of it, is less flexible than left and slightly painful.")

2. **Back of thighs (hamstrings) and calves:** Face a wall, standing two to three feet away. Bend forward and place your hands on the floor with your fingertips touching the base of the wall. With the legs straight and head tucked in, rest your upper back against the wall, keeping your heels on the ground (you should look like an upside-down V). Hold for thirty seconds.

If you have any back problems, try the easy version instead. Using a flight of stairs, put toes against the bottom step. Bend forward and place your elbows, arms crossed, on the third or forth step. If the stretch is too easy, try it on the second step instead. If there are no stairs accessible to you, use a chair. Just bend forward by placing your elbows, arms crossed, on the chair.

Evaluation: _____

(Example: "Left back of thigh, lower one-third area, plus calf are less flexible than right.")

3. **Front of chest:** Stand with your back to a wall, your heels six to eight inches from the baseboard, your knees bent slightly, and your feet hip-width apart. Lean against the wall with your shoulders, arms, and buttocks. Make sure that your lower back is not overarched. Keeping your arms against the wall, raise them straight out to your sides until they are parallel with the floor. Bend your elbows to a 90-degree angle and rest the backs of your wrists flat against the wall, with fingers pointing up. Hold for thirty seconds.

Evaluation : _____

(Example: "Left front of chest is stiff, cannot touch forearm on the wall, and wrist is not flat against the wall. My back is also arching.")

If these three stretches cause pain and discomfort, introduce the flexibility program described below and then reevaluate your flexibility regularly by doing the above three stretches. Comfort, correct posture, and symmetry of flexibility between the right and left sides are critical. Inflexibility not only creates muscles imbalances around the core but could put you at greater risk for injuries, such as torn ligaments, muscle strains, and arthritis. It's important to stretch regularly.

Active-Isolated Stretching

The active-isolated stretching technique for your neck, chest, torso, back, buttocks, and leg muscles has recently been discovered to be the best and most efficient way to stretch, based on techniques developed by Jim and Phil Wharton (1996). With this new method of stretching, each active stretch is held for no more than two seconds and repeated ten times. The old-fashioned method of stretching requires holding a stretch for thirty seconds and repeating each stretch once or twice. You can apply either of these two techniques. It is a matter of personal preference.

Jim and Phil Wharton say that to actively stretch, contract one group of muscles, so the opposing group will reflexively lengthen. For instance, to stretch the back of your thigh muscles (hamstrings), contract the front of your thigh muscles (quadriceps). To do this, lie on your back, bend one knee while the other leg (the leg you are stretching) stays straight. Take a beach towel and hold the ends together so that it forms a loop. Place the foot of the leg you are stretching into the loop. From your hip, and using the front of your thigh muscles, lift your leg up. Aim your foot toward the ceiling. When the back of your thigh muscles feel loose, you are ready to stretch your leg. Take the stretch to the limit of the leg's range of motion, that is, until you can stretch it no further. Then give yourself a gentle extra assist. Use your towel to pull your leg. Hold that new stretch for two seconds and repeat it for ten consecutive repetitions, reaching further every time. Repeat the stretch with the other leg.

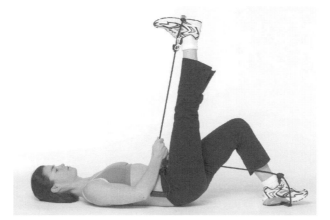

To stretch the front of the thigh, lie on your side with your knees against your chest in a fetal position. With your bottom hand, hold your bottom foot stationary. With your upper hand, grasp your upper foot. Contract the back of your thigh muscles and move your upper leg back as far as you can go. Use your hand to give an extra assist at the end of the stretch. If you cannot reach your foot with your hand, use a towel, wrapping it around the ankle of your stretching leg. Repeat with the other side.

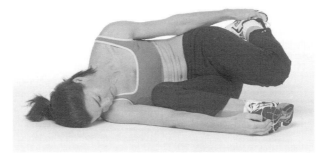

Use this method for all the other major muscle-group pairs, as follows.

Abdominal (Oblique)/Lower Back (Erector Spinae)

To stretch the abdominals, kneel down or sit in a chair with your back straight and with your feet resting on the floor. Bend forward and put your hands behind your neck with your elbows pointing outwards. Contract your lower back muscles as you rotate and extend your torso in one direction until you have twisted as far as you can go. When you feel loose, after five repetitions in one direction, return to an upright position and do the opposite side.

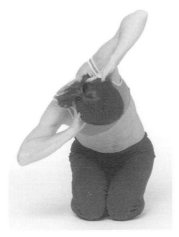

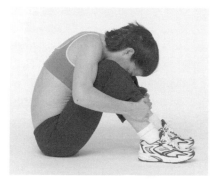

To stretch the lower back muscles, sit on the floor or in a chair with your back straight, your knees bent, and your feet resting on the floor. Tighten your abdominal muscles to pull your body forward into a slouch position. Hold the sides of your lower legs with your hands to assist at the end of the stretch.

Hip Flexor (Iliopsoas)/ Hip Extensor (Gluteal)

To stretch the front muscles of the hip (hip flexor), position yourself on your hands and knees. Reach back with the right hand to hold your right ankle. Contract the back of your right thigh and buttock muscles as you lift the leg up until the thigh is parallel to the floor or aligned horizontally with your body. Do not arch your back. Use your right hand to gently assist at the end of the stretch. Repeat with the other side.

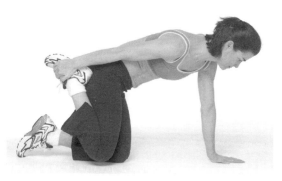

To stretch the back muscles of the hip (hip extensor), lie flat on your back with both legs straight out. Contract your abdominal and hip flexor muscles as you lift the left leg up. Place the left hand on the back of the left knee as you bend it. The right hand reaches for the right ankle as you twist the lower leg toward the right. You can give extra assistance by rotating the lower leg further toward the right shoulder. Repeat with the other side.

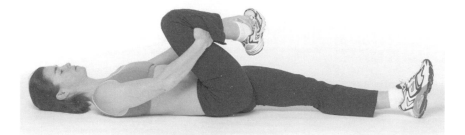

Chest (Pectorals)/ Mid Back (Rhomboids)

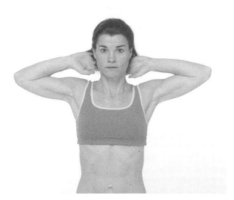

To stretch the chest, place your hands behind your neck and touch your elbows in front of your face. Pull your elbows back as far as they can go as you contract the muscles in the middle of your back. You can give extra assistance by taking a deep breath in.

To stretch the muscles in the middle of your back, stand with your feet slightly apart and your arms at your side. Lift the right arm with the elbow straight and raise it across your chest toward the left shoulder. Use the left hand to give a gentle assist at the right elbow at the end of the movement. Keep your torso stationary. Repeat with the other side.

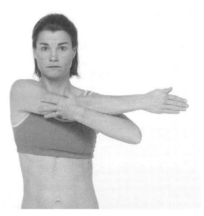

Neck Lateral Flexor (Upper Trapezius)/ Neck Extensor (Cervical Paraspinals)

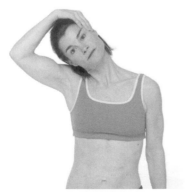

To stretch the neck lateral flexor muscles, kneel down or sit in a chair with your back straight and your feet flat on the floor. Look straight ahead. Bend your head to the right side by grasping your left ear with your right hand and pull very gently to the right to assist the end of the movement. Make sure that you keep your shoulders down and your body straight. Repeat with the other side.

To stretch the neck extensor muscles, kneel down or sit in a chair with your back straight and your feet flat on the floor. With your hands placed on the back of your head, pull your head forward until your chin touches your chest. You can assist the end of the movement by letting gravity pull your head further down toward the floor. Make sure that you keep your shoulders down and your body straight.

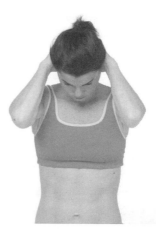

As you work on flexibility, always remember to stretch both sides. By doing so, you will probably notice if one side is less flexible than the other; you will be able to tell if you have less range of motion on one side. If so, then the goal over time is to reach a balance of flexibility between the two sides. You can achieve this balance of flexibility by stretching the less flexible side with a few more repetitions (such as twelve versus ten repetitions).

Getting Started

Get active your way, every day, and for life. Physical activity does not have to be very hard; it just has to be built into your daily routine. Starting slowly is safe for most people. You will customize your workout by first basing it on your muscle strength and then advancing at your own pace to more challenging levels. If you are unsure about this program, consult with your health professional before beginning.

Generally, the workouts should take only twenty minutes of your day. If you cannot devote twenty minutes of your day, four to seven times a week, life is very much in control of you, instead of you being in control of your life. So start today, and be in control of your life.

The Solid to the Core muscular strength program starts in chapter 2 with five series of static pelvis stabilization exercises (see table 1 of chapter 2) to give your body a solid foundation. Chapters 3 and 4 then introduce the dynamic pelvis stabilization exercises (table 2 of chapter 3) and the Swiss ball stabilization exercises (table 3 of chapter 4).

To ensure safety and readiness, the natural progression for core training is to go from a static stabilization position to a dynamic one. You need to create a stable base of support statically from the abdomen, hips, and lower back muscles before you can transfer energy to your arm and leg muscles dynamically. This energy transfer is an important ingredient for daily activities, such as gardening, raking leaves, carrying groceries, walking distances, dancing, or any sports that require running faster, throwing further, or jumping higher.

Once you master the basics, you will incorporate multiple planes of motion (moving your body from right to left in space) or different load amounts (weights) into the program. Think of it as building your own house. First you build the foundation (the core), then the walls and roof (the arms and legs and the head), and later, you might add a two-car garage. It's important to train the core as an anchor in a variety of spinal positions and motions that reflect normal, everyday postures.

Analyzing Your Muscular Strength

This program should be useful to you whether you have exercised all your life or are just starting out. To get started, you will first need to determine your current muscular strength, using the "ab plank" exercise below. Or if you already have been doing some core strength exercises, you may be able to determine your strength based on how often you have been doing them. Once you have determined your muscular strength, you can then begin to customize your workout by choosing the corresponding level of difficulty: beginner, intermediate, or advanced. (Refer to table 1 in chapter 2, which outlines the first five series of exercises.)

Ab Plank Exercise

Kneel on the floor with forearms resting on the floor. Make sure your elbows are in line with your shoulders and that your knees are behind your hips. Keep your head and neck aligned with your spine. Balancing on your toes and forearms, lift your knees two to four inches off the floor so that your body weight is equally distributed as you hold your body straight (like a plank of wood) for as long as you can.

Beginner level: If you hold the ab plank position for less than thirty seconds, if you have never done core exercises before, if you have not exercised in three or more months, or if you are recovering from an injury, you should start at the beginner level (see row one in table 1).

Intermediate level: If you can hold the ab plank position for thirty to sixty seconds or if you have been doing core strength exercises twice a week for at least three months, start at the intermediate level (see row three in table 1).

Advanced level: If you can hold the ab plank position for more than sixty seconds or if you have been doing core strength exercises three times a week for at least six months, start at the advanced level (see row four in table 1).

Progressing Through the Exercises

Notice that the exercises in each series advance in difficulty as you move vertically down each column in table 1. Level 1 is row one (exercise 1 in each series), level 2 is row two (exercise 2 in each series), level 3 is row three (exercise 3 in each series), and so on. You will start on the level most appropriate for you and gradually progress through each series of exercises, using the following protocols, as you develop greater muscle strength.

Static Pelvis Stabilization Protocol

If you are at the beginner level 1, do the corresponding row of five exercises in table 1 every other day. This means you will be doing exercise 1 in each series (A through E). Likewise, if you are starting at intermediate level 3, start with exercise 3 in each series. Complete one set of eight to ten repetitions, resting thirty to forty-five seconds between each exercise. When you can do one set of ten repetitions comfortably, add a second set.

If you are at the advanced level 4, you can do four to seven sessions a week, once or twice daily. Complete two sets of eight to ten repetitions of the five exercises in the series in table 1, resting thirty to forty-five seconds between each exercise.

At the end of one week, evaluate your progress. Note that evaluations of your progress should always occur after seven days. As a rule, you will not advance to the next level of any exercise partway through a week; progressions must always be made a week apart. Some of the exercises will be easier than others to master, depending on your own muscle imbalances and the level of difficulty. In order to advance to the next level in a series, you should find the exercises that you were doing the previous week relatively easy. Read the descriptions and attempt the next level of exercises in the series (the higher-numbered exercises in the next row down). If an exercise in one series presents a challenge but can be done in a slow and controlled manner with little if any movement of the core, you should advance to the next level. If the next level is too difficult, however, you must remain at the previous exercise level for another full week.

Note that you may advance in one series while remaining at the same level in another. As an example, in week two you might find that exercise A-1 is easy to do. If that is the case, move ahead to exercise A-2. However, exercise B-1 might still be difficult to perform, so you would continue doing it for another full week. If C-1 is easy, progress to C-2, and so on. At the beginning of week two, your exercise program could be: A-2, B-1, C-2, D-2, E-1. You can record your progress on the chart that follows each protocol.

Dynamic Pelvis Stabilization Protocol

Table 2 of chapter 3 lists the four dynamic series (F through I). After four weeks—or once you are at level 5 or 6 of the exercises in table 1 of chapter 2—and you feel you have developed a strong base of your core, you can start table 2. Once you are ready to start, add F-1. Evaluate your progress at the end of the week, and if F-1 is easy to do, you can increase the level of difficulty by moving on to F-2. At the end of the following week, you could move on to F-3, and so on, vertically down the column. Remember to keep doing the exercises in A through E until you reach the bottom of each series.

After you have successfully completed the F series, you can combine these exercises with the G series to increase your challenge. You do not need to complete the G series in any particular order, but instead, simply try out different pairs of F-G exercises together. As an example, one day you might do exercise F-1 combined with G-1 and the next day, you might do F-1 with G-2 or F-1 with G-3, and so on. By then, you should have six exercises to do, five from series A through series E and one exercises from the F and G series combined. Continue to work on the F-G paired exercises until you feel comfortable with a variety of combinations. Remember to evaluate your progress at the end of each week.

Refer to table 2 of chapter 3. You can introduce the H series once you have mastered the F-G combinations. Again, evaluate yourself at the end of each full week. You should have six exercises, five from series A through series E and one from the H series. Once you have completed each exercise of the H series, introduce the I series one at a time. Again you should have six exercises to do, five from series A through series E and one from series I.

Swiss Ball Stabilization Protocol

The J series through L series progress differently from the other series. Refer to table 3 of chapter 4. Begin by performing exercises 1 through 6 in the first column (J series). After working four to six weeks on the J series, stop doing it and progress to the intermediate K series and master that series for another four to six weeks. Once you've mastered the K series, attempt the advanced L series. These series may take you longer to advance in than the static and dynamic stabilization series. This is only natural, as the exercises are more demanding. The Swiss ball stabilization program may be continued indefinitely as a maintenance program. However, if you want to take on another very challenging protocol, refer to table 4 of chapter 5. The resistance band stabilization protocol will not only give you the "solid" balanced muscles foundation that you have been fine-tuning all along throughout this program, but will also give you the great sculpted abs that you have been dreaming of all your life.

Resistance Band Stabilization Protocol

The M series through O series progress similarly to the Swiss ball stabilization protocol. Refer to table 4 of chapter 5. You start by performing exercises 1 through 5 in the beginner column (M series). After four to six weeks on the M series, progress to the intermediate N series and master that series for another four to six weeks. After mastering that series, attempt the advanced O series.

Correct Postural Alignment

As you do each of these exercises, keep your hips parallel with your shoulders. You should imagine the spine, the hips, and the shoulders as a single unit. This stable unit should be maintained during each exercise even if the rest of the body is in motion. Do not hold your breath while doing the exercises; inhale and exhale with normal depth and rhythm. Another key requirement for completing the exercises in this program is to find your neutral position and do an abdominal set.

The *neutral position* is achieved by doing the following:

1. Lie down with your knees bent, torso aligned, arms at each side, and chin at a 90-degree angle.

2. Curve your lower spine a few times up toward the ceiling (convexity) and down toward the floor (concavity) until you find a position of comfort for your spine. This position of comfort is your spine's neutral and balanced position. Everyone's neutral position is unique.

Once you have found that neutral and balanced position, you can go on to do an *abdominal set*. To do this, you activate your abdominal muscles by pulling your navel slightly inward toward your spine, creating a flattening or a concavity of your stomach (not of your back). You can use your fingers to feel your abdomen contract. If you have difficulty activating those deep abdominal muscles, imagine your stomach as being a huge marshmallow. As you press with your fingers slightly down on the marshmallow (your stomach), the marshmallow will form a concavity, increasing in density and spreading vertically and horizontally. This analogy resembles what you will feel when you do an abdominal set. Your stomach will have a slight concavity, your back will be denser, and your spine will decompress. Do not hold your breath and do not contract your gluteal muscles. The set is strictly abdominal.

The abdominal set is the first exercise in the static pelvis stabilization A series. It is important that you master this exercise, as you are required to do it throughout the program. You will begin each exercise by finding your neutral position and doing an abdominal set.

Equipment Needed

A major advantage of the Solid to the Core strength exercise program is that it requires so little prefabricated equipment and you can do it in the comfort of your home. You will need the following items:

- **cushion:** Any kind, shape, and/or size will do.

- **small beach ball or medicine ball:** Balls can be weighted or not. They should be easily gripped and durable. You can buy them in a package of three of varying weights.

- **elastic band:** Elastic resistance materials are available in several grades or thicknesses. The thicker the elastic material, the greater the resistance. If you decide to attempt the exercises in chapter 5, you will need to purchase the Bally Total Fitness Pilates 4-way Ab Stretch.

- **wobble board:** This can be constructed simply by balancing a piece of three-quarter-inch plywood, or a flexible yet durable wooden board, on top of a wooden dowel. Wobble boards are also sold at many fitness stores.

- **step/stairs:** Any steps, stools, or stairs will do, but be sure to inspect them carefully to make sure they are safe. Avoid stairs with protruding nails or rotten or cracked wood surfaces.

- **floor mat:** You can use any type of padded mat or rug, instead of doing the exercises directly on the floor. This is suggested mainly for comfort.

- **bench:** If you do not have a bench, you can use a table, a piano bench, a bed, an ottoman, or even the top of your stairs with your legs hanging down over the stairs. What will not do is a chair or a bench with a back or arms on it.

- **free weights:** These are graduated weights that are hand held or applied to the upper or lower extremity and can be barbells, dumbbells, cuff weights with velcro closures, sandbags, and/or weight boots. You can even use cans from your kitchen cupboard.

- **Swiss ball:** To select a Swiss ball of the appropriate size, consult the following chart:

Ball Diameter	Your Height
45 cm	up to five feet (1.5m)
55 cm	from five to five-foot-six (1.5m to 1.7m)
65 cm	from five-foot-seven to six feet (1.7m to 1.8m)
75 cm	above six feet (1.8m)

Lifestyle Tips

The Solid to the Core program should be part of a healthy lifestyle that includes regular exercise. Maintaining this program as part of a comprehensive workout regime will result in a healthier and stronger back, neck, and spine.

Many of us have difficulty maintaining a fitness program due to many factors, including not having enough time, or procrastination due to stress, low energy, and the expectation of immediate results. You may have frustrating moments, agonizing over whether you will be able to pick up the kids on time from school or over what you will cook for dinner. You may wince at a twinge in your neck and you feel overwhelmed, choosing to relax in front of the TV when you finally have some downtime. If this sounds familiar, you are one of thousands of people whose hectic lifestyle leads to symptoms that may not be recognized for what they are: signs of stress, poor nutrition, or injuries.

You can help your body and mind cope more effectively with stress, and achieve greater balance in your life, if you can find the time and energy for a regular exercise program. A daily hit of aerobic exercise will release endorphins, which will give you the power to make better decisions and help you be at peace with yourself. It will also help keep you healthy, since stress can be a contributing factor to many illnesses.

Note: If you are dealing with an injury, be alert to any signs and symptoms that you may encounter. Consult a physician before beginning any exercise program.

Injuries can be prevented. It is up to you to exercise with intelligence and to be always in pursuit of better nutrition, better rest, and better exercise protocols. Pay attention to warning signs, such as muscles tightness and soreness, muscle cramping, achiness, fatigue, and joint pain. Warning signs can vary every time you exercise, so be extra careful if you have any kind of cardiovascular or musculoskeletal injuries. The body can start to compensate if something is not working properly, which will cause muscle imbalances and possibly result in more injuries.

Diet often suffers when life is hectic, but what you eat has a significant effect on how you heal and how you feel. Good nutrition can improve your ability to handle stress and can prevent injuries. Many nutritionists recommend that carbohydrates should provide 65 percent, fats 20 percent, and proteins 15 percent of your caloric intake.

Avoid buying processed or take-out foods. There are plenty of ways to make your meals appealing and suitable for your lifestyle. Have a healthy breakfast every morning that includes grains, fruits, and some proteins. Drink a lot of water throughout the day; a hydrated body fights fatigue. Say no to caffeine and sweets that have temporary energy boosts, as well as to trans-fatty fast food that has minimal nutritional value. Trans fat is a health issue, but so is the total amount of fat you eat. Next time you ask yourself, "Do I want potato chips, french fries, or doughnuts?" reach for a fruit or veggie! With healthy food in your body, you will have more energy to exercise properly, you will feel less stress, and you will recover more quickly from injuries.

CHAPTER 2

Static Pelvis Stabilization

TABLE 1: Static Pelvis Stabilization

Series A	Series B	Series C	Series D	Series E
Dead Bug	Sit-Ups	Bridging	Prone/Quadruped	Static Stabilization
Stimulates deep abdominal flexors (transversus abdominis)	Stimulates superficial abdominal flexors (rectus abdominis and obliques)	Stimulates gluteus muscles co-contracting with transversus abdominis	Stimulates deep extensor paraspinals (multifidus)	Stimulates series A, B, C, D simultaneously in space
1 Abdominal Set	Half-fold	Hip lateral rotation	Prone straight leg raise	Forward lean in sitting position
2 Hook-lying extremity flexion	Obliques	Bridging	Prone opposite arm and leg lift	Forward lean in half-kneeling position
3 Hook-lying bent leg lift	The fold	Bridging with bilateral hip flexion	Hip extension unilateral/arm lift	Backward lean in sitting position with arm lift
4 Hook-lying combination	Lower abs	Bridging with foot lift	Hip extension bilateral	Backward lean in kneeling position with arm lift
5 Hook-lying heel walk	Double knee lift	Bridging with knee extension	Quadruped lower extremity extension	Backward extension/ glute-lumbar stabilizers
6 Straight leg raise	The V position	Bridging with straight leg raise	Quadruped opposite upper/lower extremity extension	Advanced backward extension/ glute-lumbar stabilizers
7 Advanced straight leg raise	Ab plank	Ab plank with straight leg raise	Push-up/ unilateral hip extension	Back rotation in standing position from above and below

General Guidelines

Frequency: four to seven times per week

Set(s): one to two per day

Repetitions: eight to ten per exercise

Number of exercises: five (one in each series)

Reevaluation of series A through series E for progression of exercises: at the end of each week

Weekly Evaluation

| Date | Table 1
Static Pelvis Stabilization
Series A-B-C-D-E | | | | | Table 2
Dynamic Pelvis Stabilization
Series F-G-H-I | | | |
	Series A Dead Bug	Series B Sit-Ups	Series C Bridging	Series D Prone/ Quadruped	Series E Static Stabilization	Series F Lower Extremity	Series G Upper Extremity	Series H Functional Drills	Series I Plyometrics
Example: 7/15/ 2006	A #1	B #1	C #1	D #1	E #1				
7/21/ 2006	A #2	B #1	C #2	D #2	E #1				

After four weeks into the static pelvis stabilization exercises, you can begin to introduce the dynamic pelvis stabilization exercises, found in table 2. Once you have mastered all the static and dynamic exercises, you can stop doing them and move on to the Swiss ball stabilization exercises, found in table 3.

Static A Series: Dead Bug

Exercise 1 – Abdominal Set

- Lie on your back. Knees bent, feet flat on floor. Find neutral position.

- Pull belly button toward spine, flattening abdomen outwards (like you are being cinched by a corset). Pressing the navel to the spine is very often confused with sucking in the stomach, which will make you hold your breath. Instead, think of a weight attached to your navel from the inside and pulling it down and out. This action will engage your core muscles and help protect your lower back. Hold for five seconds. Release.

- Repeat.

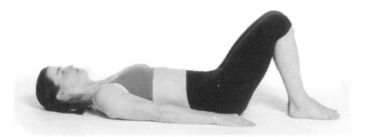

Note: *Do not tighten your neck or buttock muscles. The movement is strictly abdominal with no tilting of the pelvis. It is not a pelvic tilt. Remember to breathe.*

Exercise 2 – Hook-Lying Extremity Flexion

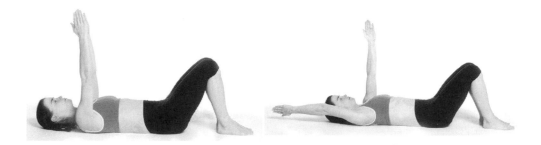

- Lie on your back. Knees bent, feet flat on floor. Lift arms over chest. Find neutral position. Do an abdominal set, as per exercise 1.

- Lower one arm overhead. Keep arm straight at the elbow. Hold for five seconds. Slowly return to starting position.

- Repeat, alternating arms.

Note: *Do not allow your back to arch.*

Variation: Slowly, holding a small ball in your hands, lower both arms overhead. Repeat.

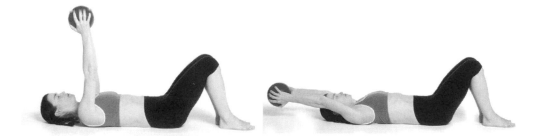

Exercise 3 – Hook-Lying Bent Leg Lift

- Lie on your back. Knees bent, feet flat on floor. Relax your arms at your side with palms down. Find neutral position. Do an abdominal set.

- Slowly raise one leg so that knee and hip are bent to 90 degrees. Hold for five seconds. Then slowly lower your leg to starting position.

- Repeat, alternating legs.

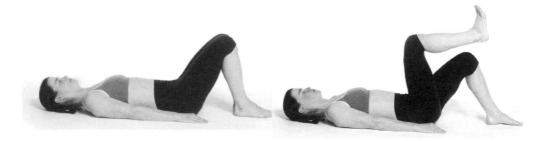

Note: *To help prevent movement of the pelvis when lifting your foot off the floor, try to make your foot weightless without actually moving it. Once it feels as though it is unweighted you should have already made the necessary muscular adjustments to be able to lift it up without pelvic movement.*

Do not allow your back to arch.

Variation: Outstretch arm (on the same side as the knee raised) to the raised knee. Push your hand and knee against each other for five seconds with 5 percent of the total force you can exert, keeping arm straight. Slowly return arm and leg to starting position.

Repeat, alternating sides.

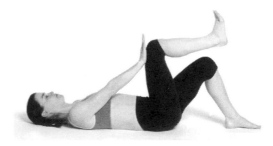

Exercise 4 – **Hook-Lying Combination**

- Lie on your back. Bend right hip and knee to 90 degrees, keeping your left foot on the floor. Lift arms to 90 degrees over chest with small ball in hands, elbows straight. Find neutral position. Do an abdominal set.

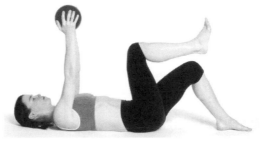

- Slowly lower your right leg to the floor, keeping knee bent at 90 degrees. Simultaneously lower both arms overhead, keeping elbows straight, until the ball is approximately one inch off the floor. Hold for five seconds. Slowly return to starting position.

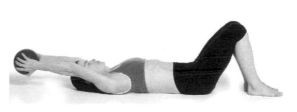

- Repeat, alternating legs.

Note: *Do not allow your back to arch.*

Exercise 5 – Hook-Lying Heel Walk

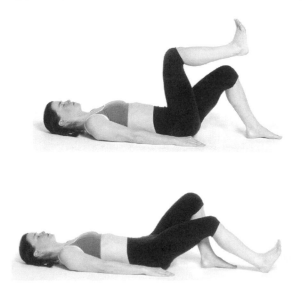

- Lie on your back. Bend right hip and knee to 90 degrees, keeping your left foot on the floor. Relax your arms at your side with palms down. Find neutral position. Do an abdominal set.

- Slowly walk right heel away from pelvis in short steps until your leg is straight. When your leg is straight, your foot should be one inch off the floor. Hold for five seconds. In the same manner, slowly return to starting position.

- Repeat, alternating legs.

Note: *Do not allow your back to arch.*

Variation: Slowly walk heel away from pelvis in short steps until leg is straight. Simultaneously lower both arms overhead with small ball in hands. Hold for five seconds. Slowly return to starting position.

Repeat, alternating legs.

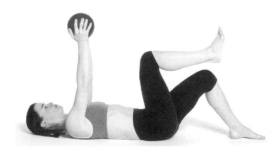

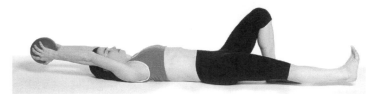

Exercise 6 – Straight Leg Raise

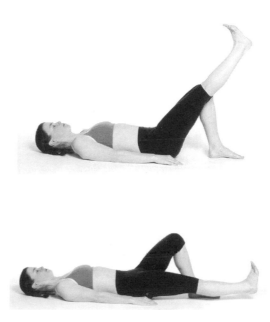

- Lie on your back. Left knee bent, left foot flat on the floor. Right hip bent to 45 degrees with knee straight, so that right and left thighs are in line. Relax arms at your side with palms down. Find neutral position. Do an abdominal set.

- While keeping your knee straight, slowly lower your right leg parallel to one inch above the floor. Hold for five seconds. Slowly return to starting position.

- Do half of the repetitions on one side; change legs and complete the remainder of the repetitions.

Note: *Do not allow your back to arch.*

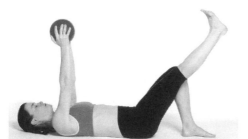

Variation: Slowly lower your leg until it is one inch above the floor, keeping knee straight. Simultaneously lower both arms overhead with small ball in hands, keeping elbows straight. Hold for five seconds. Slowly return to starting position.

Do half of the repetitions on one side; change legs and complete the remainder of the repetitions.

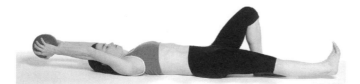

Exercise 7 – Advanced Straight Leg Raise

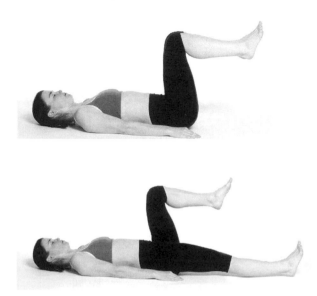

- Lie on your back. Bend both hips and knees to 90 degrees. Relax arms at your side with palms down. Find neutral position. Do an abdominal set.

- Slowly straighten right leg from the knee and hip until it is one inch from the floor, keeping knee straight. Hold for five seconds. Slowly return to starting position.

- Repeat, alternating legs.

Note: *Do not allow your back to arch.*

Variation 1: Slowly straighten right leg from the knee and hip until it is one inch from the floor. Simultaneously lower both arms overhead with small ball in hands, keeping elbows straight. Hold for five seconds. Slowly return to starting position.

Repeat, alternating legs.

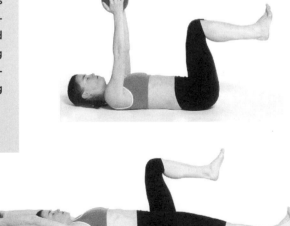

Variation 2: Clasp your hands behind your neck. Slowly straighten left leg from the knee and hip until it is one inch from the floor. Simultaneously rotate your upper body to the right, keeping elbows in line with shoulders. (You may put weight on your right shoulder.) Hold for five seconds. Slowly return to starting position.

Repeat, alternating sides.

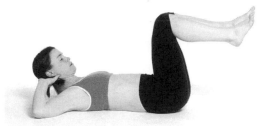

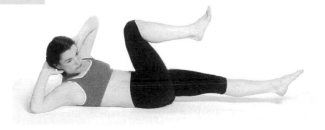

Static B Series: Sit-Ups

Exercise 1 – Half-Fold

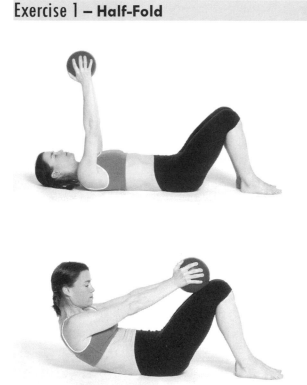

- Lie on your back. Knees bent, feet flat on floor. Lift arms to 90 degrees over chest with small ball in hands, elbows straight. Find neutral position. Do an abdominal set.

- Lift upper body (one vertebra at a time) into a crunch as your arms extend forward and reach with the small ball toward knees; shoulder blades should clear the floor. Keep your upper body lifted and arms straight. Hold for five seconds. In the same manner, slowly return to starting position.

- Repeat.

Variation: Lift upper body (one vertebra at a time) into a crunch as your arms extend forward and reach with the small ball toward knees; shoulder blades should clear the floor. Keep your upper body lifted and arms straight. Slowly raise the small ball overhead and return it to your knees. Slowly lower your body one vertebra at a time to starting position.

Repeat.

Exercise 2 – Obliques

- Lie on your back. Left knee bent, foot flat on floor. Rest your right ankle on your left thigh and let your right knee fall to the outside. Clasp hands behind neck (not head) with elbows in line with shoulders and resting on the floor. Find neutral position. Do an abdominal set.

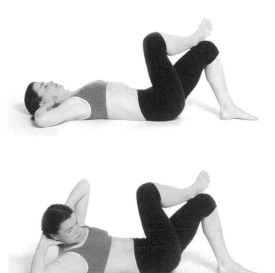

- Lift head and shoulders off floor while rotating as one unit to the right side until your left shoulder blade is just off the floor. Keep elbows in line with shoulders. Hold for five seconds. Slowly return to starting position.

- Do half of the repetitions on one side; change sides and complete the remainder of the repetitions.

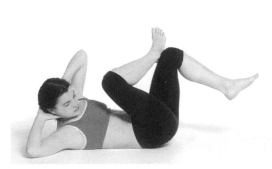

Variation: Lift head and shoulders off floor while rotating as one unit to the right side until your left shoulder blade is just off the floor. Simultaneously raise left leg off the floor as you rotate your upper body to the right. Hold for five seconds.

Do half of the repetitions on one side; change sides and complete the remainder of the repetitions.

Exercise 3 – The Fold

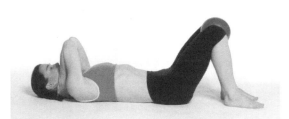

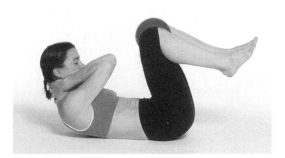

- Lie on your back. Knees bent, holding the small ball between them, feet flat on floor. Clasp hands behind neck (not head) with elbows pointing toward the ceiling. Find neutral position. Do an abdominal set.

- Lift upper body (one vertebra at a time) into a crunch until your shoulder blades are just off the floor. Simultaneously curl hips off the floor bringing knees toward elbows. Hold for five seconds. Slowly return to starting position.

- Repeat.

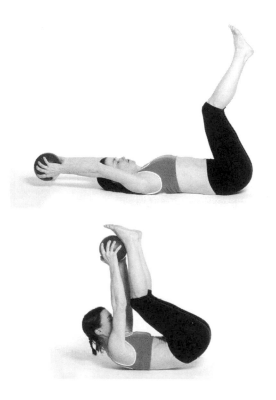

Variation: Lie on your back. Arms overhead with the small ball between your hands, keeping your elbows straight. Hips bent at 45 degrees from your upper body, knees bent so feet are in line with hips. Find neutral position. Do an abdominal set.

Lift upper body (one vertebra at a time) into a crunch, lifting the small ball overhead, keeping elbows straight. Simultaneously curl hips off the floor bringing knees toward elbows. Continue to curl until the small ball is in contact with your ankles. Hold for five seconds. Slowly return to starting position.

Repeat.

Exercise 4 – Lower Abs

- Lie on your back. Bend hips and knees to 90 degrees, holding the small ball between your knees. Elbows bent at 90 degrees, in line with shoulders. Relax forearms on floor with palms up. Find neutral position. Do an abdominal set.

- Curl buttocks off the floor keeping upper body, shoulders, arms, and neck on the floor. Hold for five seconds. Slowly lower buttocks to starting position.

- Repeat.

Note: *Do not let your legs rock back and forth as momentum. If it happens, hold the leg of your couch with both hands for stability of your torso.*

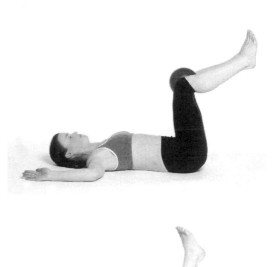

Exercise 5 – Double Knee Lift

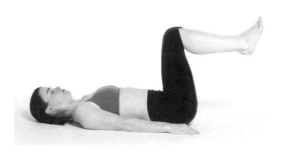

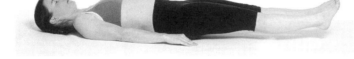

- Lie on your back. Both hips and knees bent to 90 degrees. Relax arms at your side with palms down. Find neutral position. Do an abdominal set.

- Slowly straighten both legs from the hip and the knee until they are one inch above the floor. Hold for five seconds. Slowly return to starting position.

- Repeat.

Note: *Do not allow your back to arch.*

Variation: Slowly straighten both legs from the hip and the knee until they are one inch above the floor. Simultaneously lower both arms overhead with small ball in hands, keeping elbows straight. Hold for five seconds. Slowly return to starting position.

Repeat.

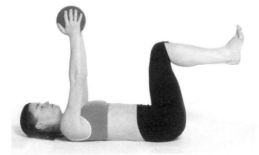

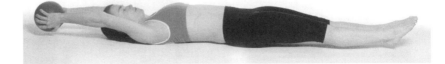

Exercise 6 – The V Position

- Sit on the floor. Bend hips and upper body to 90 degrees. Bend knees to 45 degrees holding the small ball between them with feet off the floor. Bend elbows to 90 degrees with hands flat on the floor, fingers pointing forward. Find neutral position. Do an abdominal set.

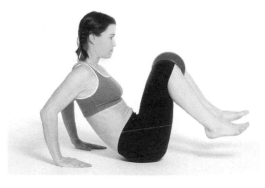

- Slowly extend your knees so that your legs are straight at 45 degrees from the floor. Simultaneously bend elbows so that your upper body is at a 45-degree angle from the floor, keeping upper body straight. Hold for five seconds. Slowly return to starting position.

- Repeat.

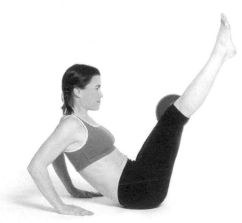

Note: *Try to use stomach muscles instead of arms to hold upper body in position.*

Exercise 7 – Ab Plank

- Kneel on the floor with forearms resting on floor. Elbows in line with shoulders and knees slightly behind your hips. Hold the small ball between your knees. Keep head and neck aligned with spine. Find neutral position. Do an abdominal set.

- Lift knees two to four inches off the floor so that body weight is equally distributed over forearms and toes, holding the body straight (like a plank of wood). Hold for five seconds. Slowly return to starting position, keeping knees just above the floor.

- Repeat.

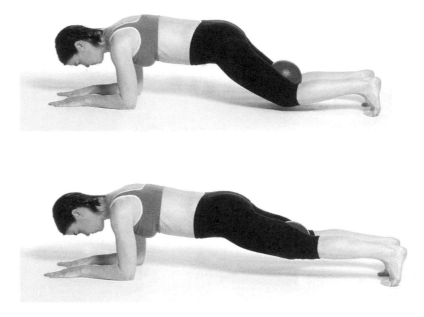

Static C Series: Bridging

Exercise 1 – Hip Lateral Rotation

- Lie on your right side. For more support, position yourself against a wall. Bend hips and knees to 90 degrees. Holding the small ball in your hands, rest arms on the floor over your head, keeping elbows straight. Find neutral position. Do an abdominal set.

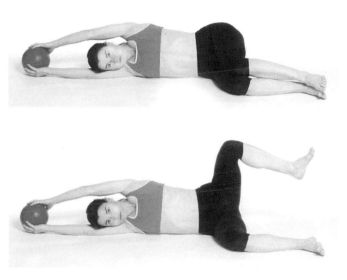

- Using buttock muscles, slowly rotate left hip outward, pointing knee and foot to the ceiling. Keep pelvis in line with torso. Hold for five seconds. Slowly lower left hip to starting position.

- Do half of the repetitions on one side; change sides and complete the remainder of the repetitions.

Note: *Do not allow your back to arch.*

Variation: Tie a resistance band around knees.

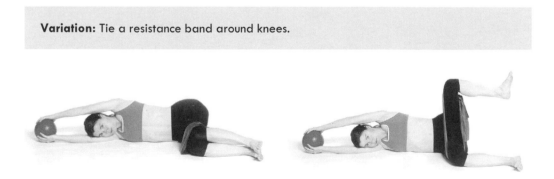

Exercise 2 – Bridging

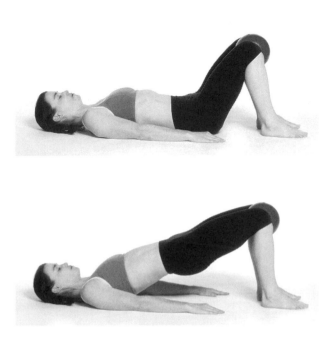

- Lie on your back. Knees bent, feet flat on floor. Hold the small ball between your knees. Find neutral position. Do an abdominal set.

- Using buttock muscles, slowly raise pelvis from floor, keeping trunk rigid. Make sure that you do not do a pelvic tilt to raise hips or arch back to raise torso higher. Relax shoulders and neck. Hold for five seconds. Slowly return to starting position.

- Repeat.

Note: *If hamstrings are tight, move feet closer to buttocks. Think of pushing your knees out over your feet to lift pelvis without tilting. You should be moving only through the hip joint, not the waist.*

Exercise 3 – Bridging with Bilateral Hip Flexion

- Lie on your back. Knees bent, feet flat on floor. Hold the small ball between your knees. Find neutral position. Do an abdominal set.

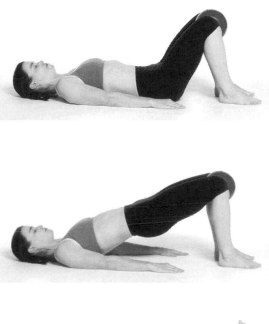

- Using buttock muscles, slowly raise pelvis from the floor, keeping trunk rigid. Hold for five seconds. Slowly return to starting position. Slowly flex both hips to 90 degrees, keeping trunk rigid. Hold for five seconds. Slowly return to starting position.

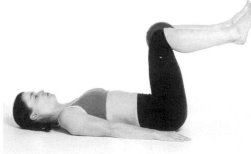

- Repeat by alternating between raising your pelvis and flexing both hips.

Exercise 4 – Bridging with Foot Lift

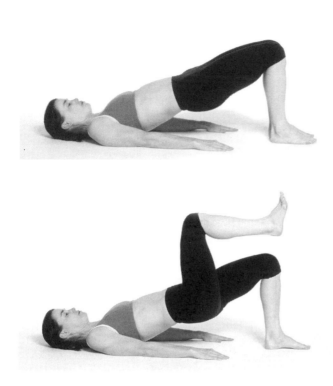

- Lie on your back. Knees bent, feet flat on floor. Find neutral position. Do an abdominal set.

- Using buttock muscles, slowly raise pelvis from the floor, keeping trunk rigid until pelvis is in line with knees and shoulders. Flex your right hip and knee to 90 degrees, without moving your pelvis, keeping your trunk rigid. Hold for five seconds. Slowly return to starting position.

- Repeat, alternating legs.

Note: *Placing a stick across your hips will help you to maintain the stabilization of your pelvis. The stick should not dip to one side or roll off.*

Exercise 5 – Bridging with Knee Extension

- Lie on your back. Knees bent, feet flat on floor. Find neutral position. Do an abdominal set.

- Using buttock muscles, slowly raise pelvis from the floor, keeping trunk rigid until pelvis is in line with knees and shoulders. Slowly extend right leg from the knee without moving your pelvis, keeping trunk rigid, until leg is straight. Both thighs should remain at the same level. Hold for five seconds. Slowly return to starting position.

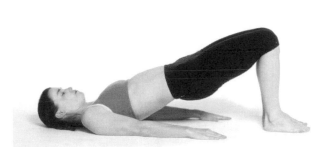

- Repeat, alternating legs.

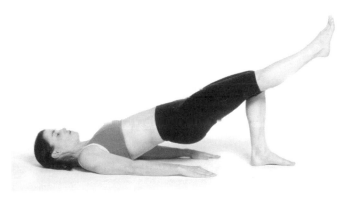

Note: *Placing a stick across your hips will help you to maintain the stabilization of your pelvis. The stick should not dip to one side or roll off.*

Exercise 6 – Bridging with Straight Leg Raise

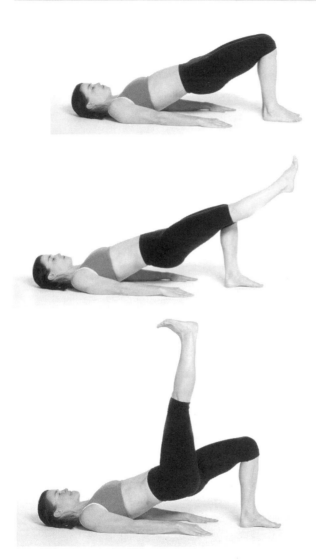

- Lie on your back, knees bent, feet flat on floor. Find neutral position. Do an abdominal set.

- Using buttock muscles, slowly raise pelvis from the floor, keeping trunk rigid until pelvis is in line with knees and shoulders. Slowly extend right leg from the knee like a hinge, until leg is straight, keeping thighs in line. Flex right hip to your maximum hamstring flexibility (keeping knee straight bring leg as far as possible toward head) without moving your pelvis, while keeping trunk rigid. Hold for five seconds. Slowly return to starting position.

- Do half of the repetitions on one side; change legs and complete the remainder of the repetitions.

Exercise 7 – Ab Plank with Straight Leg Raise

- Position yourself face up with your knees bent at 90 degrees, feet flat on floor. Hands should be directly under shoulders, fingers facing forward. Find neutral position. Do an abdominal set.

- Using buttock muscles, slowly raise pelvis from the floor, keeping trunk rigid until pelvis is in line with knees and shoulders, so that you are balancing on your palms and feet and looking forward. Then slowly extend one leg from the knee until the leg is straight and parallel to upper body. Flex hip to 45 degrees without moving your pelvis, keeping the trunk rigid. Hold for five seconds. Slowly return to starting position.

- Do half of the repetitions on one side; change legs and complete the remainder of the repetitions.

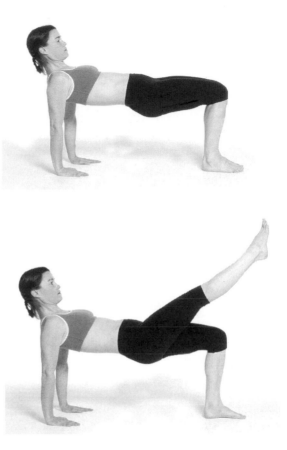

Static D Series: Prone/Quadruped

Exercise 1 – Prone Straight Leg Raise

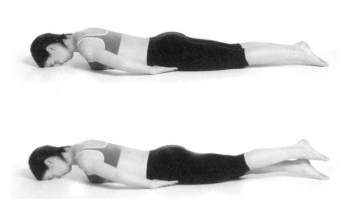

- Lie on your stomach. Place your hands under your pelvis bones. Place a tightly rolled towel under your forehead to keep neck and spine aligned. Find neutral position. Do an abdominal set.

- Straighten left knee. Slowly raise left leg two to four inches off the floor while tightening buttock muscles. Feel that you are stretching your leg toward the wall behind you, instead of the ceiling above you. Keep your pelvis bones in touch with hands, putting symmetrical pressure on both sides. Hold for five seconds. Slowly return to starting position.

- Repeat, alternating legs.

Note: *Do not allow your back to arch. You can put a pillow under your pelvis and hips, should you feel that it would help.*

Variation: Bend left knee to 90 degrees. Slowly raise thigh one to two inches off the floor using buttock muscles. Hold for five seconds. Slowly return to starting position.

Do half of the repetitions on one side; change legs and complete the remainder of the repetitions.

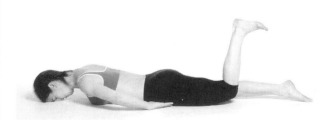

Exercise 2 – Prone Opposite Arm and Leg Lift

- Lie on your stomach. Outstretch arms overhead on the floor, palms down. Place a tightly rolled towel under your forehead to keep neck and spine aligned. Find neutral position. Do an abdominal set.

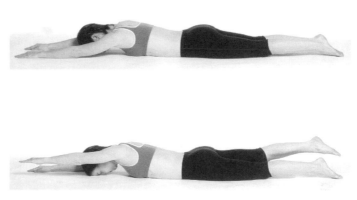

- Slowly raise right leg one to two inches off the floor, using your buttock muscles. Simultaneously lift your left arm one inch off the floor. Feel that you are stretching in opposition, fingers and toes reaching for the opposite walls of the room (not for the ceiling). Do not move pelvis or shoulders; only the limbs should move. Hold for five seconds. Slowly return to starting position.

- Repeat, alternating arms and legs.

Note: *Do not allow your back to arch. You can put a pillow under your pelvis and hips, should you feel that would help.*

Exercise 3 – Hip Extension Unilateral/Arm Lift

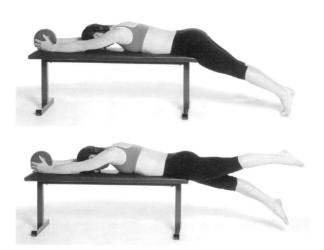

- Lie face down on a bench with your hips resting against the edge of the bench. (If you do not have a bench, see page 20 for suggestions about what to use instead.) Place a tightly rolled towel under your forehead to keep neck and spine aligned. Outstretch arms overhead on the table holding the small ball between your hands. Rest feet on the floor. Find neutral position. Do an abdominal set.

- Using buttock muscles, slowly raise left leg until it is parallel to the floor. Keep pelvis bones on the bench with symmetrical pressure on both sides. Hold for five seconds. Slowly return to starting position.

- Repeat, alternating legs.

Note: *Do not allow your back to arch. Do not push off the floor with the foot that is remaining on the floor; it should remain relaxed.*

Variation 1: Using buttock muscles, slowly raise left leg until it is parallel to the floor. Simultaneously raise right arm one inch off the table.

Repeat, alternating arms and legs.

Variation 2: Using buttock muscles, slowly raise left leg until it is parallel to the floor. Begin to raise right leg. Legs should meet at 45 degrees and cross like scissors. Continue until the right leg is parallel to the floor and the left leg is resting on the floor.

Repeat, alternating legs.

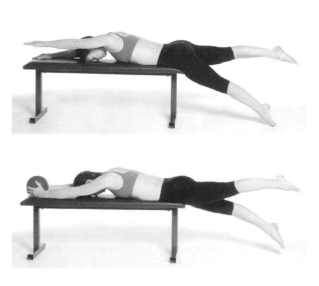

Exercise 4 – Hip Extension Bilateral

- Lie face down on a bench with your hips resting against the edge of the bench. (If you do not have a bench, see page 20 for suggestions about what to use instead.) Place a tightly rolled towel under your forehead to keep neck and spine aligned. Out-stretch arms overhead on the bench, holding the small ball between your hands. Rest feet on the floor. Find neutral position. Do an abdominal set.

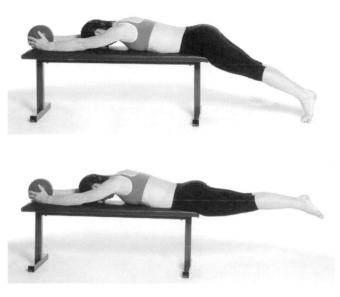

- Using your buttock muscles, slowly raise both legs until they are parallel to the floor. Keep your pelvis bones on the bench with symmetrical pressure on each side. Hold for five seconds. Slowly return to starting position.

- Repeat.

Note: *Do not allow your back to arch.*

Exercise 5 – Quadruped Lower Extremity Extension

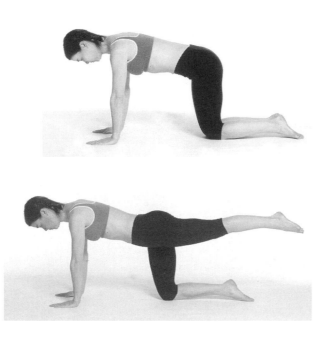

- Kneel on the floor hands on the floor, under shoulders, knees under hips. Keep spine straight and head aligned with spine. Find neutral position. Do an abdominal set.

- Maintaining upper body alignment, slowly slide left leg along the floor until it is straight. Then using buttock muscles, lift left leg until it is parallel with ground. Feel that you are stretching your leg toward the wall behind you instead of the ceiling above you. Keep pelvis and shoulders level. Hold for five seconds. Slowly return to starting position, keeping trunk rigid.

- Repeat, alternating legs.

Note: *Do not allow your back to arch or to flex.*

Exercise 6 – Quadruped Opposite Upper/Lower Extremity Extension

- Kneel on the floor, hands on the floor under shoulders, knees under hips. Keep spine straight and head aligned with spine. Find neutral position. Do an abdominal set.

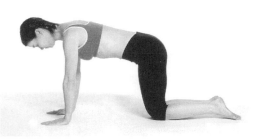

- Maintaining upper body alignment, slowly slide left leg along the floor until it is straight. Then, using buttock muscles, lift left leg until it is parallel with ground. Simultaneously, slowly slide

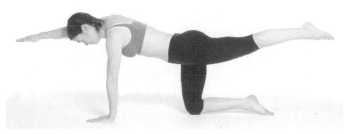

right hand forward until arm is straight and lift right arm until it is parallel with the floor. Stretch in opposite directions, fingers and toes reaching for opposing walls of the room. Hold for five seconds. Slowly return to starting position, keeping trunk rigid.

- Repeat, alternating legs and arms.

Note: *Do not allow your back to arch or to flex.*

Exercise 7 – Push-Up/Unilateral Hip Extension

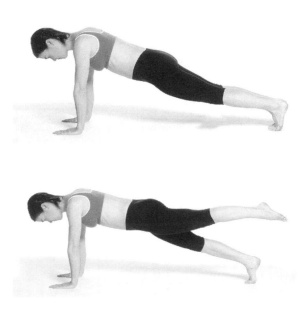

- Begin in push-up position. Hands directly beneath shoulders and legs together, standing on your toes. Your body should be as a plank, in line from your shoulders to your toes. Keep neck long and head aligned with your spine. Find neutral position. Do an abdominal set.

- Point your left foot. Using your buttock muscles, raise left leg until it is parallel to the floor. Hold for five seconds. Slowly return to starting position, keeping trunk rigid.

- Repeat, alternating legs.

Note: *Do not allow your back to arch. Keep a flat body from your head to heels.*

Variation: Point your left foot. Using your buttock muscles, raise left leg until it is parallel to the floor. Simultaneously bend elbows in a push-up. Hold for five seconds when two inches from the floor. Slowly return to starting position.

Repeat, alternating legs.

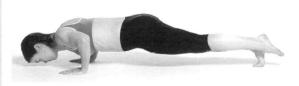

Static E Series: Stabilization

Exercise 1 – Forward Lean in Sitting Position

- Sit at the edge of a chair. Hold the small ball between your knees. Bend both the hips and the knees at 90 degrees. Chin should be at 90 degrees so that ears are in line with shoulders and shoulder blades are pulled down and inwards toward the spine. Find neutral position. Do an abdominal set.

- Keep body in a lengthened position as though someone were pulling a string attached to your vertebrae. Lean forward at the hips to about 45 degrees. Hold for five seconds. Slowly push back from the feet to return to starting position, keeping trunk rigid.

- Repeat.

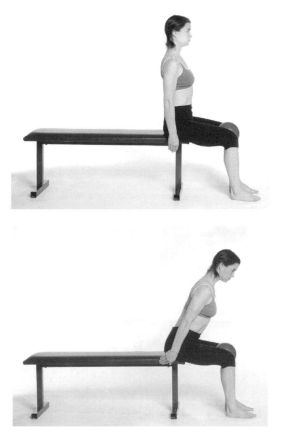

Note: *There should be no movement of your waist or shoulders. The only movement should be a hinge forward from the hips.*

Exercise 2 – Forward Lean in Half-Kneeling Position

- Kneel with right leg forward, and front knee bent to 110 degrees. Chin should be at 90 degrees so that ears are in line with shoulders and shoulder blades are pulled down and inwards toward the spine. Hold the small ball in your hands with your arms behind your back, keeping elbows straight. Find neutral position. Do an abdominal set.

- Keeping shoulders in line with the left knee, move right knee forward over toes. Hold for five seconds. Slowly return to starting position, keeping trunk rigid and pushing back with right leg, not using your torso.

- Do half the repetitions with the right leg; kneel with the left leg forward, and complete the remaining repetitions.

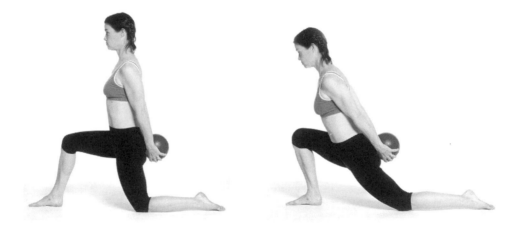

Note: *Do not allow your back to arch or flex. The body moves as a unit; there should be no bending at the waist or shoulders.*

Exercise 3 – Backward Lean in Sitting Position with Arm Lift

- Sit at the edge of a chair. Hold the small ball between your knees. Bend knees to 110 degrees. Chin should be at 90 degrees so that ears are in line with shoulders and shoulder blades are pulled down and inwards toward the spine. Focus on a point directly in front of you. Find neutral position. Do an abdominal set.

- Keep body in a lengthened position as though someone were pulling a string attached to your vertebrae. Slowly recline your upper body from the hips until the upper body is at a 45-degree angle from the chair. Hold for five seconds. Slowly return to starting position, keeping trunk rigid.

- Repeat.

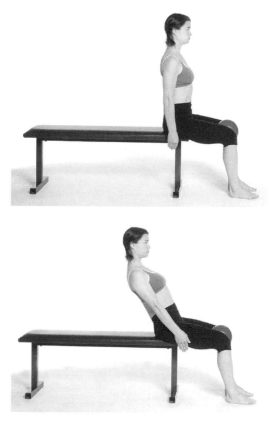

Note: *Do not allow your back to arch or bend.*

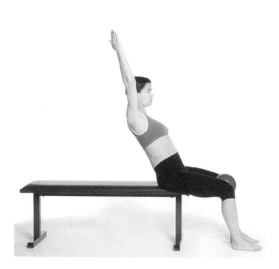

Variation: Keep body in a lengthened position as though someone were pulling a string attached to your vertebrae. Slowly recline your upper body from the hips until it is at a 45-degree angle from the chair. Raise right arm until it is in line with your ears. When it is in line with your ears, begin to raise left arm. Arms should meet at 90 degrees and cross like scissors. Continue until the left arm is in line with ears and the right arm is in line with your upper body at hips.

Raise each arm once and slowly return to starting position, keeping trunk rigid. Repeat.

Exercise 4 – Backward Lean in Kneeling Position with Arm Lift

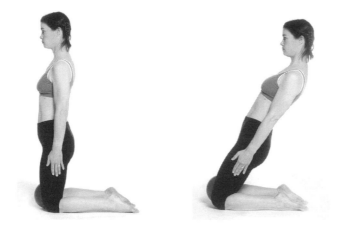

- Kneel on both knees. Hold the small ball between your knees. Chin should be at 90 degrees so that ears are in line with shoulders and shoulder blades are pulled down and inwards toward the spine. Focus on a point directly in front of you. Find neutral position. Do an abdominal set.

- Keep body in a lengthened position as though someone were pulling a string attached to your vertebrae. Slowly recline from the knees to 45 degrees from the floor, keeping your upper body as a unit from the knees to the shoulders. Hold for five seconds. Slowly return to starting position, keeping trunk rigid.

- Repeat.

Note: *Do not allow back to arch or bend.*

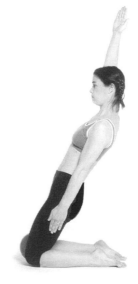

Variation: Keep body in a lengthened position as though someone were pulling a string attached to your vertebrae. Slowly recline from the knees to 45 degrees from the floor, keeping your upper body as a unit from the knees to the shoulders. Raise right arm until it is in line with your ears. When it is in line with your ears, begin to raise left arm. Arms should meet at 90 degrees and cross like scissors. Continue until the left arm is in line with ears and the right arm is in line with your upper body at hips.

Raise each arm once and slowly return to starting position, keeping trunk rigid.

Repeat.

Exercise 5 – Backward Extension/Glute-Lumbar Stabilizers

- Lie facedown on the floor with legs straight behind you. Place a tightly rolled towel under your forehead to keep neck and spine aligned. Hold the small ball on the small of your back, keeping your chest and shoulders down. Find neutral position. Do an abdominal set.

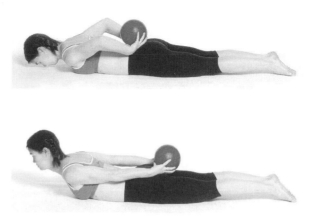

- Keeping legs straight, tighten buttocks. Lift upper body off the floor and slide the small ball further down your back until arms are fully extended. Hold for five seconds. Slowly return to starting position.

- Repeat.

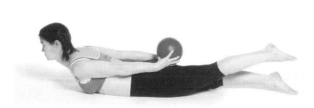

Variation 1: Keeping legs straight, tighten buttocks. Lift upper body off the floor and slide the small ball further down your back until arms are fully extended. Simultaneously lift left leg one to two inches off the floor. Hold for five seconds. Slowly return to starting position.

Repeat, alternating legs.

Variation 2: Keeping legs straight, tighten buttocks. Lift upper body off the floor and slide the small ball further down your back until arms are fully extended. Simultaneously lift both legs one to two inches off the floor. Hold for five seconds. Slowly return to starting position.

Repeat.

Exercise 6 – Advanced Backward Extension/Glute-Lumbar Stabilizers

- Lie with legs resting on a table so that your hip bones are at the edge of the bench and your upper body extends beyond the bench. Cross your arms over your chest holding the small ball against the chest, keeping body parallel to the floor. Brace your feet under an immovable object or have someone hold your ankles. Find neutral position. Do an abdominal set.

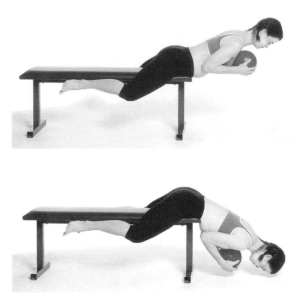

- Slowly bend downward to 45 degrees. Keep body in a lengthened position as though someone were pulling a string attached to your vertebrae. Hold for five seconds. Slowly return to starting position, keeping trunk rigid.

- Repeat.

Note: *Do not allow your back to arch or flex.*

Variation: Without the small ball, keep upper body straight and parallel to the floor. Hold left arm forward so that it is parallel with the floor in line with your ears; hold the right arm parallel to the floor in line with your hips. Slowly bring arms toward each other so that they cross like scissors perpendicular to the floor and continue so that your right arm is in line with your ears and your left arm is in line with your hips, keeping trunk rigid.

Repeat, alternating arms until each arm has been in line with ears ten times.

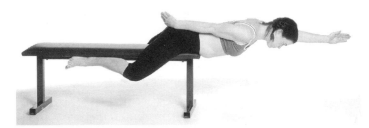

Exercise 7 – Back Rotation in Standing Position from Above and Below

- Stand with your knees hip-width apart and slightly bent. Place one end of a resistance band under one foot and the other end between your hands. Find neutral position. Do an abdominal set.

- Keep body in a lengthened position as though someone were pulling a string attached to your vertebrae. Slowly bend forward at the hips. Rotate and side-flex

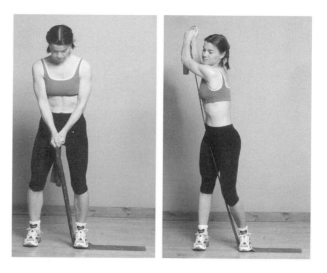

upper body and head away from the resistance band until back is extended. (This is a similar motion to a golf swing follow-through). Hold for five seconds. Slowly return to starting position, keeping trunk rigid.

- Do half the repetitions rotating to one side. Complete the repetitions rotating to the other side.

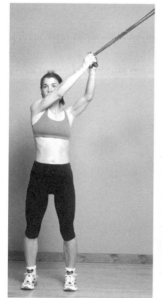
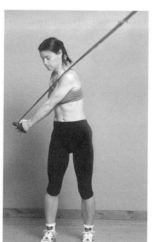

Variation: Attach one end of the resistance band to the top of a closed door. Pull it down and across your upper body toward the floor, keeping trunk rigid.

Do half of the repetitions pulling toward your right foot; complete the remainder of the repetitions facing the other way so that you are pulling toward your left foot.

CHAPTER 3

Dynamic Pelvis Stabilization

TABLE 2: Dynamic Pelvis Stabilization

Series F	Series G	Series H	Series I
Lower Extremity Patterns	Upper Extremity Patterns	Functional Drills	Plyometrics
1. Wall slide	1. Flexion-extension pattern	1. Squat with balance board	1. Squat jumps
2. Squats	2. Diagonal pattern	2. Single leg squat on step	2. Split squat jumps
3. Static lunges	3. Compression/axial loading	3. Static lunges with cushion	3. Standing long jumps
4. Dynamic lunges	4. Static core recruitment antagonist contraction (CRAC)	4. Dynamic lunges with step	
	5. Dynamic core recruitment antagonist contraction (CRAC)		

General Guidelines

Frequency: four to seven times per week

Set(s): one to two per day

Repetitions: eight to ten per exercise

Number of exercises: six, one in each series of A through E, plus one in series F later combined with G series

Reevaluation of series A through series F for progression of exercises: at the end of each week

When to start G series: Once the F series is completed, you can combine any of the F series with any of the G series as a new challenge.

When to start H series: Once you have mastered the combined F and G series, you can eliminate them and introduce the H series (now doing A through E, plus H).

When to start I series: Once the H series has been mastered, you can eliminate it and introduce the I series (now doing A through E, plus I).

Dynamic F Series: Lower Extremity Patterns

Exercise 1 – Wall Slide

- Stand against the wall. Chin should be at 90 degrees so that ears are in line with shoulders and shoulder blades are pulled down and inwards toward the spine. Let arms fall to the side with palms facing the wall. Place the small ball between your knees. Feet should be far enough away from the wall that when you sit with your knees bent to 90 degrees your hips are against the wall and your ankles are bent at 90 degrees. Find neutral position. Do an abdominal set.

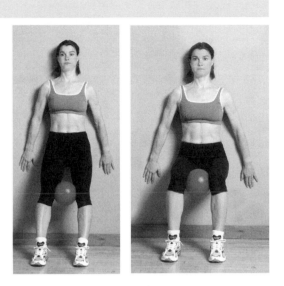

- Keeping good neutral posture, bend your knees. As you slide down the wall, maintain contact between your hips and the wall. Bend knees until you reach a knee angle of 45 to 90 degrees. Do not allow your thighs to go any lower than parallel to the floor. Hold for five seconds. Slowly return to starting position by pushing with your legs.

- Repeat.

Note: *Placing a towel between your back and the wall may help you slide.*

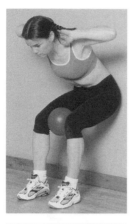

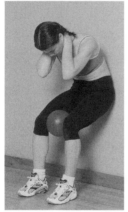

Variation: Stand with back against the wall with the small ball between your knees. Bend knees to 90 degrees, keeping hips against the wall. Extend arms overhead so that they are parallel with your ears and the palms are facing each other. Find neutral position. Do an abdominal set.

Keeping your lower and middle back firmly against the wall, round your upper torso forward and away from the wall. Visualize forming a C shape with your torso by moving one vertebra at a time. Maintaining thigh position and keeping tension on the small ball, lengthen your spine up and out into a flat diagonal line so that just your hips are against the wall. As you move, open your elbows out to the sides keeping abdominals tight. Hold for five seconds. Round your spine back to the wall to arrive at starting position.

Repeat.

Exercise 2 – Squats

- Stand with chin at 90 degrees so that ears are in line with shoulders and shoulder blades are pulled down and inwards toward the spine. Place the small ball between your knees. Find neutral position. Do an abdominal set.

- Squat until knees are bent between 45 and 90 degrees. Simultaneously, raise arms forward until they are shoulder height. Keep your body weight back on your heels and maintain abdominal set. Hold for five seconds. Slowly return to starting position.

- Repeat.

Note: *Do not allow your back to arch.*

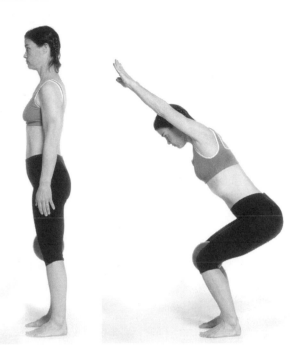

Exercise 3 – Static Lunges

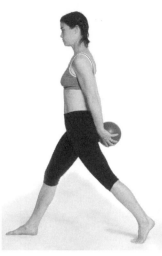

- Stand with one leg out in front of your body and the other behind. Chin at 90 degrees so that ears are in line with shoulders and shoulder blades are pulled down and inwards toward the spine. Hold the small ball in your hands behind your back. Find neutral position. Do an abdominal set.

- Lower upper body by bending the back knee to the floor. Do not allow the knee to touch the floor. Keep the hips and shoulders perpendicular to the floor at all times so there is no forward or backward motion. Slowly return to starting position, keeping trunk rigid.

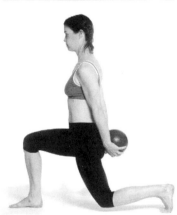

- Do half of the repetitions on one side; change legs and complete the remainder of the repetitions.

Note: *Do not allow your front knee to bend more than 90 degrees or to extend in front of the front foot.*

Variation: Stand in a wide-based stance with arms in front, holding the small ball in hands. Find neutral position. Do an abdominal set.

Shift body weight to one side, keeping shoulders horizontal, and perform a single-sided lunge. Slowly return to starting position.

Repeat, alternating legs.

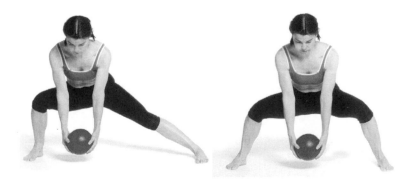

Exercise 4 – Dynamic Lunges

- Stand with feet hip-width apart. Chin at 90 degrees so that ears are in line with shoulders and shoulder blades are pulled down and inwards toward the spine. Hold the small ball in hands with arms behind your back. Find neutral position. Do an abdominal set.

- Stepping forward with right knee, lower your body down by bending the back knee to the floor. Slowly push back from the front foot to return to starting position, keeping trunk rigid.

- Repeat, alternating legs.

Note: *Do not bend your front leg more than 90 degrees or let your upper body lean forward.*

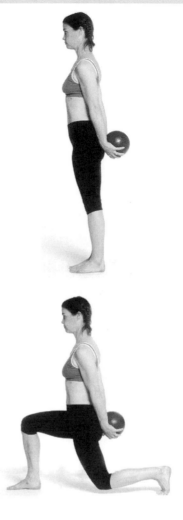

Dynamic G Series: Upper Extremity Patterns (Combined with the F Series)

Note: *As a precaution, if shoulders are injured, do not attempt these exercises.*

Exercise 1 – Flexion-Extension Pattern

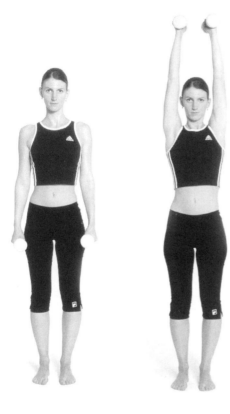

- Hold dumbbells in hands with palms facing inward and arms straight against upper thighs. Find neutral position. Do an abdominal set.

- Raise dumbbells overhead until vertical (or as far as your shoulder flexibility will allow). Lower to starting position, using same pattern.

- Combine this pattern with any of the four F-series exercises.

- Repeat.

Note: *Do not allow your back to arch.*

Exercise 2 – **Diagonal Pattern**

- Hold a dumbbell in hands with palms facing inward and arms straight in front of left thigh. Find neutral position. Do an abdominal set.

- Raise dumbbell across torso in a diagonal motion until arms are just above and parallel to right shoulder. Lower to starting position using same pattern.

- Combine this pattern with any of the four F-series exercises.

- Repeat, alternating the thigh in front of which you hold the dumbbell.

Note: *Do not allow your back to arch.*

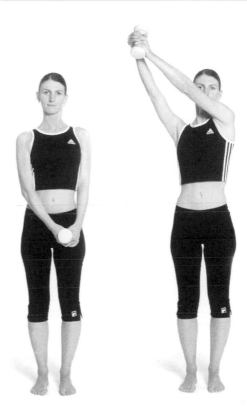

Exercise 3 – Compression/Axial Loading

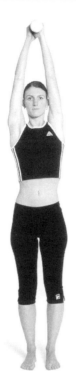

- Hold a dumbbell in hands with palms facing inward and arms straight overhead (or as far as your shoulder flexibility will allow). Find neutral position. Do an abdominal set.

- Combine this pattern with any of the four F-series exercises as you hold this position static.

Note: *Do not allow your back to arch.*

Exercise 4 – Static Core Recruitment Antagonist Contraction (CRAC)

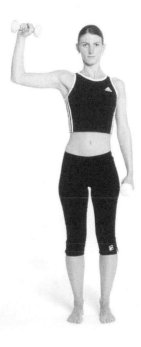

- Hold a dumbbell in each hand with arms at sides. Raise right arm until parallel to right shoulder at a 90-degree angle. Find neutral position. Do an abdominal set.

- Combine this pattern with any of the four F-series exercises as you hold this position with right arm as left arm is kept straight beside your torso.

- Do half of the repetitions on one side; change hands and complete the remainder of the repetitions.

Exercise 5 – Dynamic Core Recruitment Antagonist Contraction (CRAC)

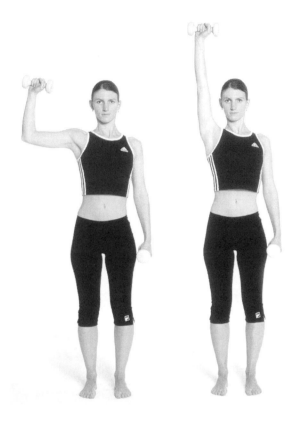

- Hold a dumbbell in each hand with arms at sides. Raise right arm until parallel to right shoulder at a 90-degree angle. Find neutral position. Do an abdominal set.

- Press dumbbell overhead until right elbow is straight as left arm is kept straight beside torso. Lower right arm to starting position.

- Combine this pattern with any of the four F-series exercises.

- Do half of the repetitions on one side; change hands and complete the remainder of the repetitions.

Note: *Do not allow your back to arch.*

Dynamic H Series: Functional Drills

Exercise 1 – Squat with Balance Board

- Place both feet on a balance board; keep head up, back straight, feet shoulder-width apart. Hold the small ball between your hands in front of your body with elbows straight. Find neutral position. Do an abdominal set.

- Squat until knees are bent between 45 and 90 degrees. Simultaneously raise arms forward. Keep your body weight back on your heels. Hold for five seconds. Slowly return to starting position, keeping trunk rigid.

- Repeat.

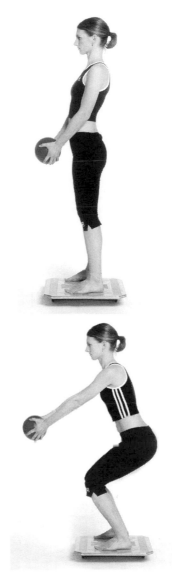

Exercise 2 – **Single Leg Squat on Step**

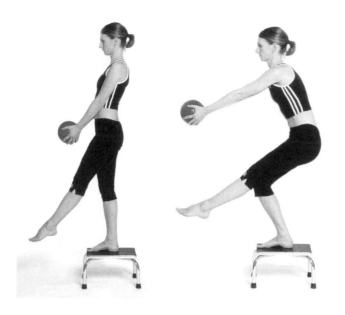

- Stand with right foot on the edge of the step and left leg hanging off the front edge of the step. Hold the small ball between your hands with arms in front of you, keeping your elbows straight. Find neutral position. Do an abdominal set.

- Drop buttocks as if you were sitting in a chair with both arms moving forward. Stop when your right thigh is between 45 degrees and parallel to the floor. Hold for five seconds. Slowly return to starting position, keeping trunk rigid.

- Do half of the repetitions on one side; change legs and complete the remainder of the repetitions.

Exercise 3 – Static Lunges with Cushion

- Stand with right leg out in front of your body and foot on a cushion. Hold the small ball between your hands with arms in front of you, keeping elbows straight. Find neutral position. Do an abdominal set.

- Lower upper body by bending your left knee to the floor without touching knee to the floor. Simultaneously raise arms forward. Hold for five seconds. Slowly return to starting position, keeping trunk rigid.

- Do half of the repetitions on one side; change legs and complete the remainder of the repetitions.

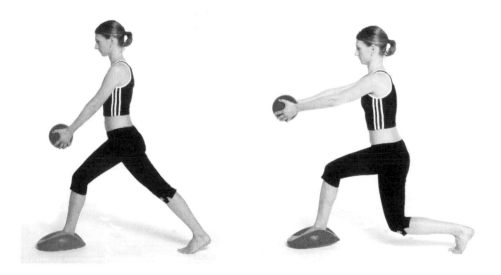

Note: *Do not allow your front knee to bend to more than 90 degrees or to extend in front of the front foot.*

Exercise 4 – Dynamic Lunges with Step

- Stand on a step with feet hip-width apart. Hold the small ball between your hands with arms behind your back, keeping elbows straight. Find neutral position. Do an abdominal set.

- Step forward onto the floor with your left leg, bending knee to 90 degrees. Lower body straight down toward the ground. Hold for five seconds. Slowly return to starting position, pushing with the left leg.

- Repeat, alternating legs.

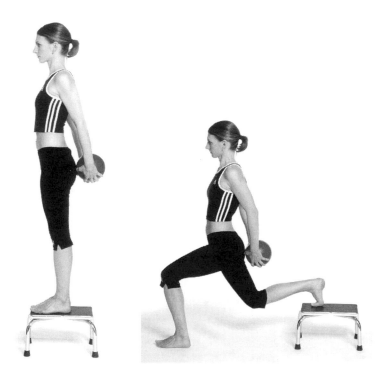

Note: *Do not let your front knee bend more than 90 degrees or let your upper body lean forward.*

Dynamic 1 Series: Plyometrics

Exercise 1 – Squat Jumps

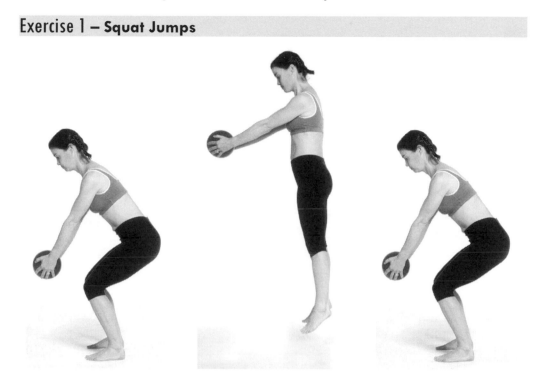

- Stand on mat or thick carpet. Start in a squat position with knees over toes, shoulder-width apart. Chin should be at 90 degrees so that ears are in line with shoulders and shoulder blades are pulled down and inwards toward the spine. Hold the small ball between your hands with arms in front of you, keeping your elbows straight. Find neutral position. Do an abdominal set.

- Jump straight up, straightening body with arms moving upwards.

- Land as softly as you can, with knees bent into squat position and keeping trunk rigid. Go right into the next jump.

Exercise 2 – Split Squat Jumps

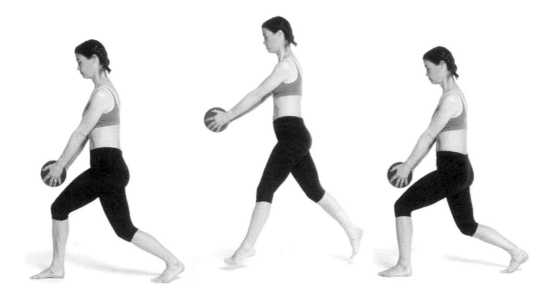

- Stand on mat or thick carpet. Start with one leg out in front of your body. The rear leg remains slightly bent. Chin should be at 90 degrees so that ears are in line with shoulders and shoulder blades are pulled down and inwards toward the spine. Hold the small ball in front of body with arms straight. Find neutral position. Do an abdominal set.

- Jump straight up, straightening body with arms moving upwards. In the air, switch legs as you prepare to land in a static lunge position, keeping trunk rigid. Go right into next jump, switching legs in the air.

Exercise 3 – Standing Long Jumps

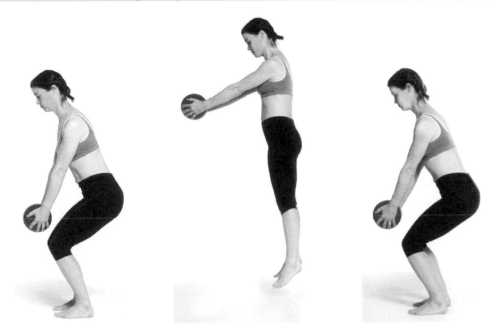

- Stand on mat or thick carpet. Start in a squat position with knees over toes, shoulder-width apart. Hold the small ball in front of body. Find neutral position. Do an abdominal set.

- Jump straight up and forward over a distance, straightening body with arms moving upwards. Land as softly as you can with knees bent into squat position, keeping trunk rigid.

- Turn around and repeat your horizontal jump

CHAPTER 4

Swiss Ball Stabilization

TABLE 3: Swiss Ball Stabilization

Series J Beginner	Series K Intermediate	Series L Advanced
1. Abdominal set in sitting position	1. Forward lean in sitting position with foot lift	1. Backward lean in sitting position with arm and leg raise
2. Half-fold with ball roll	2. Ab plank	2. The fold
3. Bridging	3. Bridging with hip flexion	3. Bridging with roll
4. Quadruped upper and lower extremity extension	4. Ab plank with unilateral hip extension	4. Push-up
5. Backward lean in sitting position	5. Back extension	5. Back extension and rotation
6. Wall slide	6. Unilateral squat	6. Lunge

General Guidelines

Frequency: four to seven times per week

Set(s): one to two per day

Repetitions: eight to ten per exercise

Number of exercises: six in the beginner series; six in the intermediate series; six in the advanced series

Reevaluation of series J–K–L: Once the J series is easy, eliminate it and introduce the K series. Do the same progressing from the K series to the L series.

Table 3		
Swiss Ball Stabilization		
Series J	**Series K**	**Series L**
Beginner	Intermediate	Advanced
Date:	Date:	Date:

In this table, just write the date of when you started the beginner series J, which you should do for up to six weeks before moving to the intermediate series K and another six weeks for the advanced.

Swiss Ball J Series: Beginner

Exercise 1 – Abdominal Set in Sitting Position

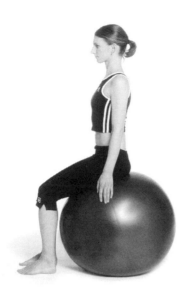

- Sit on the middle of the Swiss ball. Make sure that your weight is evenly distributed on both feet and that knees are bent to 110 degrees. Arms should hang to the side of the body. Find neutral position. Do an abdominal set.

- Hold for five seconds.

- Repeat.

Exercise 2 – Half-Fold with Ball Roll

- Lie on your back. Place your calves on the Swiss ball so that your knees are bent to 110 degrees. Hold the small ball between your hands with arms overhead and elbows straight. Find neutral position. Do an abdominal set.

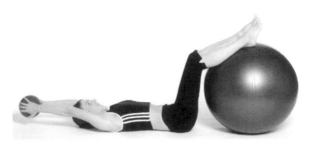

- Slowly bring arms off the floor and raise them until they are at a 45-degree angle from your body, keeping elbows locked. Curl your body one vertebra at a time while continuing to move the small ball so that it comes into

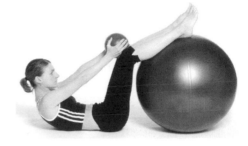

contact with knees (until shoulder blades are just off the ground). Hold for five seconds. Slowly return to starting position.

- Repeat.

Note: *Keep the chin tucked in so that your head is the last part of your body to return to the floor.*

Variation: Slowly bring arms off the floor and raise them until they are at a 45-degree angle from your body, keeping elbows locked. Curl your body one vertebrae at a time while continuing to move the small ball, reaching for the outside of the right knee (until shoulder blades are just off the ground). Hold for five seconds. Slowly return to starting position.

Repeat, alternating sides.

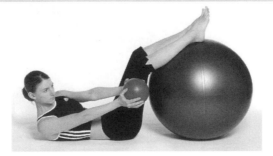

Exercise 3 – Bridging

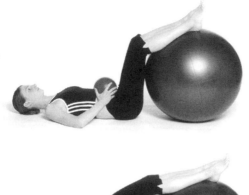

- Lie on your back. Place calves on the Swiss ball so that your knees are bent to 110 degrees. Hold the small ball on your stomach; elbows and shoulders remain relaxed. Find neutral position. Do an abdominal set.

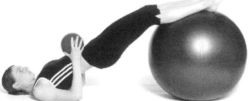

- Using buttock muscles, slowly raise pelvis from the floor, keeping trunk rigid until pelvis is in line with knees and shoulders. Hold for five seconds. Slowly return to starting position.

- Repeat.

Note: *Visualize your torso from the hip joint to your shoulders being a piece of plywood that cannot bend. Do not allow any shifting of the pelvis.*

Variation: Lie on your back. Place ankles on the Swiss ball so that your knees are straight. Hold the small ball on your stomach; elbows and shoulders remain relaxed. Find neutral position. Do an abdominal set.

Using buttock muscles, slowly raise pelvis from the floor, keeping trunk rigid until pelvis is in line with knees and shoulders. Hold for five seconds. Slowly return to starting position.

Repeat.

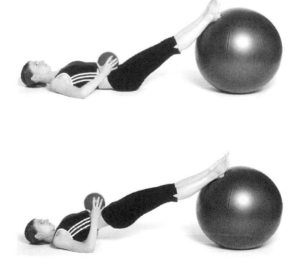

Exercise 4 – Quadruped Upper and Lower Extremity Extension

- Lie face down with pelvis on the Swiss ball. Rest hands and feet on the floor. Keep head and neck in line with spine. Find neutral position. Do an abdominal set.

- Slowly raise your right leg until it is parallel to the floor using your buttock muscles, keeping knees straight. Simultaneously raise your left arm until it is parallel to the floor, keeping elbows straight. Shoulders and pelvis should remain level. Hold for five seconds. Slowly return to starting position.

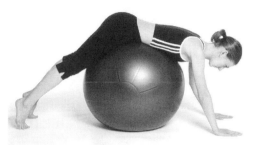

- Repeat, alternating arms and legs.

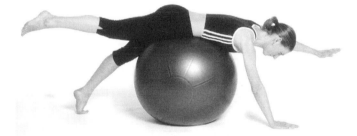

Exercise 5 – Backward Lean in Sitting Position

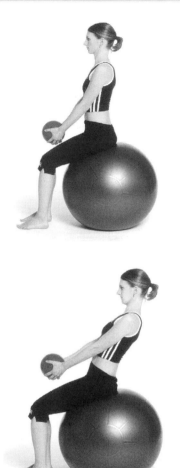

- Sit on the middle of the Swiss ball. Make sure that your weight is evenly distributed on both hips and that knees are bent to 110 degrees. Hold the small ball in your hands above your knees, keeping elbows straight. Chin should be at 90 degrees so that ears are in line with shoulders and shoulder blades are pulled down and inwards toward the spine. Focus on a point directly in front of you. Find neutral position. Do an abdominal set.

- Keep body in a lengthened position as though someone were pulling a string attached to your vertebrae. Slowly recline your upper body from the hips 45 degrees. Hold for five seconds. Slowly return to starting position, keeping trunk rigid.

- Repeat.

Variation: Keep body in a lengthened position as though someone were pulling a string attached to your vertebrae. Slowly recline your upper body from the hips 45 degrees. Keeping upper body in that position, lift the small ball overhead, keeping elbows straight. When your arms are in line with your ears, bring the small ball back, so it is over your knees. Slowly return to starting position, keeping trunk rigid.

Repeat.

Exercise 6 – Wall Slide

- Stand with your back against the Swiss ball and the Swiss ball against the wall. Hold the small ball between your knees. Chin should be at 90 degrees so that ears are in line with shoulders and shoulder blades are pulled down and inwards toward the spine. Feet should be far enough away from the Swiss ball so that when you sit with your knees bent to 90 degrees and your hips are against the Swiss ball, your ankles are at 90 degrees. Find neutral position. Do an abdominal set.

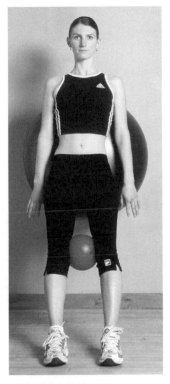

- Keeping good neutral posture, bend your knees. As you slide the Swiss ball down the wall, maintain contact between your hips and the Swiss ball. Bend knees until you reach a knee angle of 45 to 90 degrees. Do not allow your thighs to go any lower than parallel to the floor. Hold for five seconds. Slowly return to starting position by pushing with your legs, not your back.

- Repeat.

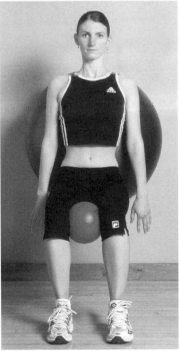

Swiss Ball K Series: Intermediate

Exercise 1 – Forward Lean in Sitting Position with Foot Lift

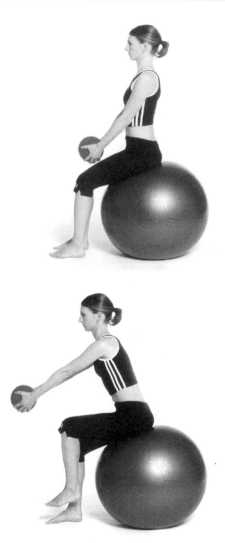

- Sit on the middle of the Swiss ball. Make sure that your weight is evenly distributed on both hips and that knees are bent to 110 degrees. Hold the small ball in your hands above your knees. Chin should be at 90 degrees so that ears are in line with shoulders and shoulder blades are pulled down and inwards toward the spine. Focus on a point directly in front of you. Find neutral position. Do an abdominal set.

- Keep body in a lengthened position as though someone were pulling a string attached to your vertebrae. Slowly lean your upper body forward 45 degrees from the hips. Raise left foot four to six inches off the floor without moving the ball. Hold for five seconds. Slowly return to starting position, keeping trunk rigid.

- Repeat, alternating legs.

Exercise 2 – Ab Plank

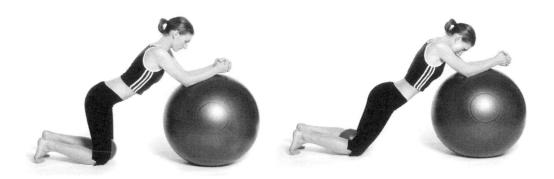

- Kneel on the floor. Thighs perpendicular to the floor, forearms resting on the Swiss ball with hands clasped. Hold the small ball between your knees. Keep head and neck aligned with spine. Find neutral position. Do an abdominal set.

- Slowly lean forward from the knees so that the Swiss ball rolls away from your body. Keep upper body in line from the hips to the shoulders. Hold for five seconds. Slowly return to starting position, keeping trunk rigid.

- Repeat.

Note: *The only movement should be through the knees and hips. Trunk remains stable.*

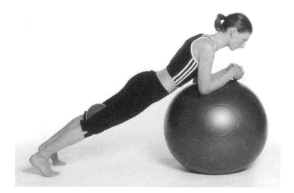

Variation: Slowly lean forward from the knees so that the Swiss ball rolls away from your body. Continue to roll the Swiss ball forward until your body is in line from your feet to your shoulders. Hold for five seconds. Slowly return to starting position, keeping trunk rigid.

Repeat.

Exercise 3 – Bridging with Hip Flexion

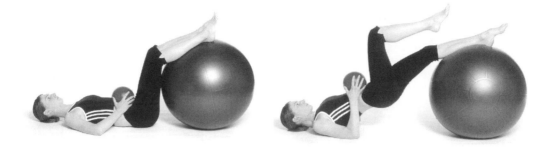

- Lie on your back. Place calves on the Swiss ball so that your knees are bent to 110 degrees. Hold the small ball on your stomach; elbows and shoulders remain relaxed. Find neutral position. Do an abdominal set.

- Using buttock muscles, slowly raise pelvis from the floor, keeping trunk rigid until pelvis is in line with knees and shoulders. Flex right hip and knee until your thigh is perpendicular to the floor. Hold for five seconds. Slowly return to starting position.

- Do half of the repetitions on one side; change sides and complete the remainder of the repetitions.

Variation: Lie on your back. Place your calves on the Swiss ball so that your knees are bent to 110 degrees. Hold the small ball between your hands with arms overhead and elbows straight. Find neutral position. Do an abdominal set.

Using buttock muscles, slowly raise pelvis from the floor, keeping trunk rigid until pelvis is in line with knees and shoulders. Flex right hip and knee until your thigh is perpendicular to the floor. Hold for five seconds. Slowly return to starting position.

Do half of the repetitions on one side; change sides and complete the remainder of the repetitions.

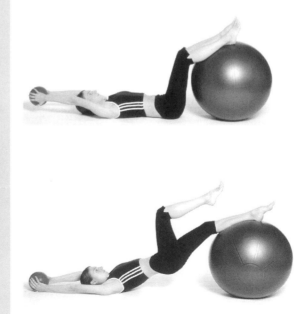

Exercise 4 – Ab Plank with Unilateral Hip Extension

- Lie with stomach on the Swiss ball. Walk forward on your hands so that your ankles are on the center of the Swiss ball. Have elbows directly under shoulders with forearms on the floor and palms facing down. Keep neck and head in line with spine. Keep body in line, from feet to shoulders. Find neutral position. Do an abdominal set.

- Using buttock muscles, raise left leg six to twelve inches off the Swiss ball. Hold for five seconds. Slowly return to starting position.

- Do half of the repetitions on one side; change sides and complete the remainder of the repetitions.

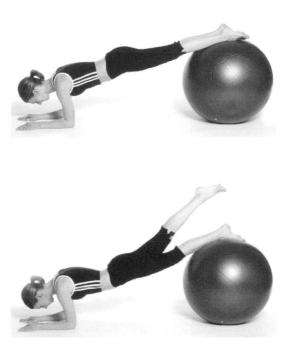

Note: Do not allow the Swiss ball to move when you are raising your leg. Do not allow hips to bend or back to arch or curl.

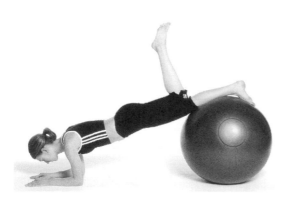

Variation: Using hamstring muscle, curl left leg toward buttocks until knee is at 90 degrees. Hold for five seconds. Slowly return to starting position.

Do half of the repetitions on one side; change sides and complete the remainder of the repetitions.

Exercise 5 – Back Extension

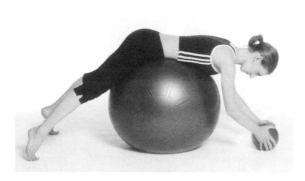

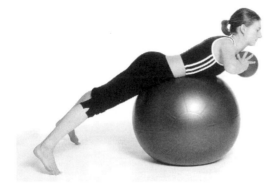

- Lie with stomach on the Swiss ball, both feet on the floor, and hold the small ball between your hands resting it on the floor. Keep neck and head in line with spine. Find neutral position. Do an abdominal set.

- Pull small ball up and into chest by bending elbows out to the side. Use back extensors to raise your chest and the small ball off of the Swiss ball. Hold for five seconds. Slowly return to starting position.

- Repeat.

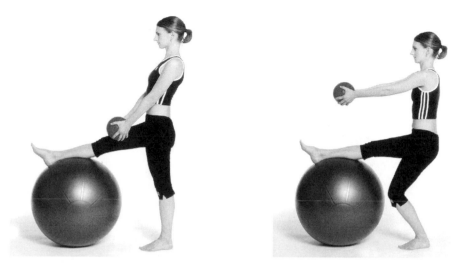

- Stand with right ankle on the center of the Swiss ball. Keep shoulders in line with the left foot. Hold the small ball in your hands over right leg, keeping elbows straight. Find neutral position. Do an abdominal set.

- Bend left knee so that your hips stay in line with your left foot. Simultaneously raise arms until they are parallel with the floor. Hold for five seconds. Slowly return to starting position.

- Do half of the repetitions on one side; change legs and complete the remainder of the repetitions.

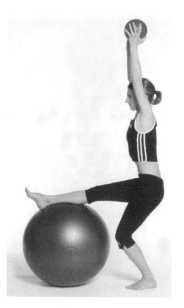

Variation: Bend left knee so that your hips stay in line with your left foot. Simultaneously raise arms until they are overhead and in line with ears. Hold for five seconds. Slowly return to starting position.

Do half of the repetitions on one side; change legs and complete the remainder of the repetitions.

Swiss Ball L Series: Advanced

Exercise 1 – Backward Lean in Sitting Position with Arm and Leg Raise

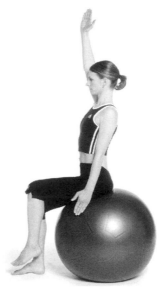

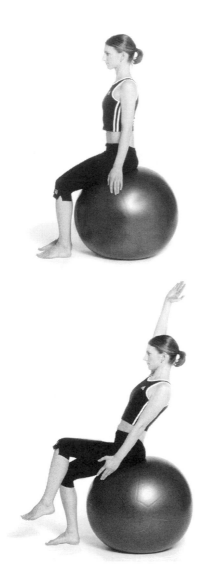

- Sit on the middle of the Swiss ball. Make sure that your weight is evenly distributed on both feet and that knees are bent to 110 degrees. Arms should hang to the side of the body. Focus on a point directly in front of you. Find neutral position. Do an abdominal set.

- Keeping the Swiss ball stable, raise left leg from the hip until your foot is one to two inches off the floor. Simultaneously raise right arm, keeping elbow straight until it is in line with your ear. Keep body in a lengthened position as though someone were pulling a string attached to your vertebrae. Slowly recline your upper body from the hips 45 degrees. Hold for five seconds. Slowly return to starting position, keeping trunk rigid.

- Repeat, alternating arms and legs.

Exercise 2 – The Fold

- Lie on your back, knees bent, feet flat on the floor. Hold the Swiss ball in your hands overhead approximately one to two inches off the floor. Keep elbows straight. Find neutral position. Do an abdominal set.

- Lift Swiss ball overhead until it is 90 degrees over chest. Continue moving the Swiss ball toward knees as you lift upper body (one vertebra at a time) into a crunch. Simultaneously curl hips off the floor bringing knees toward elbows. Continue to curl until the Swiss ball is in contact with your ankles. Hold for five seconds. Clasp Swiss ball between ankles. Uncurl hips until your pelvis is on the floor and knees and hips are at 90 degrees and the Swiss ball is held one to two inches off the floor by your feet. Do the reverse to return to starting position.

- Repeat.

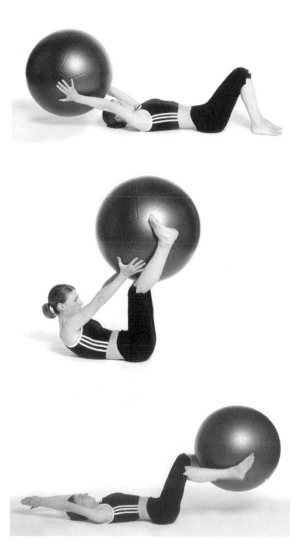

Exercise 3 – Bridging with Roll

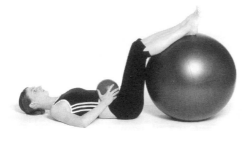

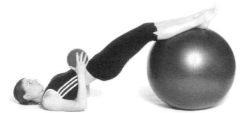

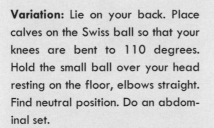

- Lie on your back. Place calves on the Swiss ball so that your knees are bent to 110 degrees. Hold the small ball on your stomach; elbows and shoulders remain relaxed. Find neutral position. Do an abdominal set.

- Using buttock muscles, slowly raise pelvis from the floor, keeping trunk rigid until pelvis is in line with knees and shoulders. Keeping trunk in line, roll the Swiss ball toward your buttocks until only your heels are on the Swiss ball. Hold for five seconds. Slowly return to starting position.

- Repeat.

Note: *Visualize your torso from the hip joint to your shoulders being a piece of plywood that cannot bend. Do not allow any shifting of the pelvis.*

Variation: Lie on your back. Place calves on the Swiss ball so that your knees are bent to 110 degrees. Hold the small ball over your head resting on the floor, elbows straight. Find neutral position. Do an abdominal set.

Using buttock muscles, slowly raise pelvis from the floor, keeping trunk rigid until pelvis is in line with knees and shoulders. Keeping trunk in line, roll the Swiss ball toward your buttocks until only your heels are on the Swiss ball. Hold for five seconds. Slowly return to starting position.

Repeat.

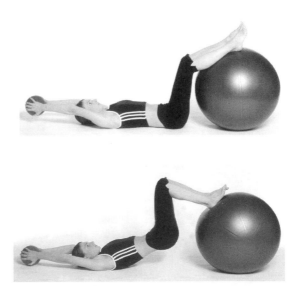

Exercise 4 – Push-Up

- Lie with stomach on the Swiss ball. Walk forward on your hands so that your ankles are on the center of the Swiss ball. Have hands directly under shoulders with fingers facing forward. Keep neck and head in line with spine. Keep body in line from feet to shoulders. Find neutral position. Do an abdominal set.

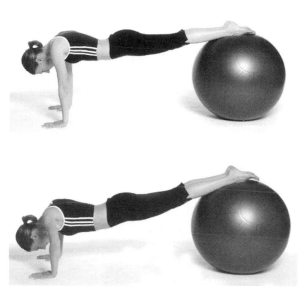

- Bend elbows until your nose is two to four inches off the floor. Keep body as a plank from the shoulders to the feet. Hold for five seconds. Slowly return to starting position.

- Repeat.

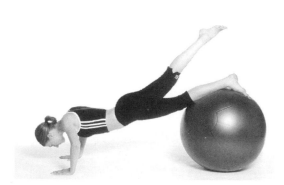

Variation: Using buttock muscles, raise left leg six to twelve inches off the Swiss ball. Simultaneously bend elbows until your nose is two to four inches off the floor. Keep body as a plank from the shoulders to the feet. Hold for five seconds. Slowly return to starting position.

Do half of the repetitions on one side; change legs and complete the remainder of the repetitions.

Exercise 5 – Back Extension and Rotation

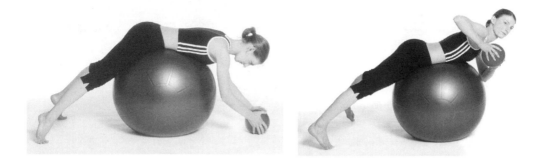

- Lie with stomach on the Swiss ball, both feet on the floor, and hold the small ball between your hands resting it on the floor. Keep neck and head in line with spine. Find neutral position. Do an abdominal set.

- Pull small ball up and into chest by bending elbows out to the side. Use back extensors to raise your chest and the small ball off of the Swiss ball. Keeping elbows and shoulders in line, rotate to the right. Hold for five seconds. Slowly return to starting position.

- Repeat, alternating sides.

> **Variation:** Lie with stomach on the Swiss ball, both hands on the floor with fingers facing forward. Hold the small ball between your knees and rest both feet on the floor. Keep neck and head in line with spine. Find neutral position. Do an abdominal set.
>
> Using buttock muscles, raise legs until they are in line with your shoulders. Rotate at the hips so that your right leg is higher than your left. Hold for five seconds. Slowly return to starting position.
>
> Repeat, alternating sides.

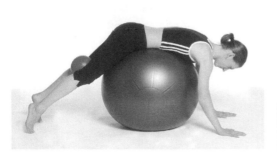
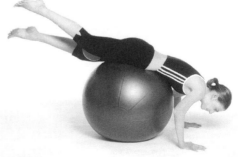

Exercise 6 – Lunge

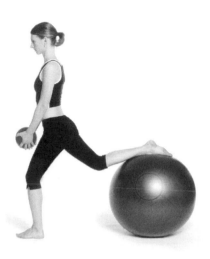

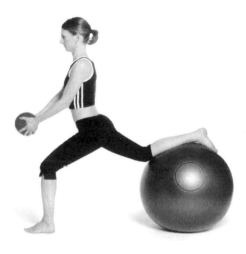

- Stand on left foot. Place right ankle on the center of the Swiss ball with leg at 45 degrees from hips. Hold the small ball in your hands over left thigh, keeping your elbows straight. Keep body in line from the hips to the shoulders. Find neutral position. Do an abdominal set.

- Slowly bend your left knee as you roll the Swiss ball backwards with your right leg. Your upper body should lower in a straight line toward the floor. Simultaneously raise your arms until they are about halfway between your thigh and parallel to the floor. Hold for five seconds. Slowly return to starting position.

- Do half of the repetitions on one side; change legs and complete the remainder of the repetitions.

CHAPTER 5

Resistance Band Stabilization

TABLE 4: Resistance Band Stabilization

Series M	Series N	Series O
Beginner	Intermediate	Advanced
1. Hook-lying combination	1. Straight leg raise	1. Double knee lift
2. Half-fold	2. The fold	2. The V position
3. Bridging	3. Bridging with knee extension	3. Bridging with straight leg raise
4. Quadruped lower extremity extension	4. Quadruped opposite upper/lower extremity extension	4. Push-up/unilateral hip extension
5. Squats with arm curls	5. Plié with front raises	5. Static lunge with one arm front raises

General Guidelines

Frequency: four to seven times per week

Set(s): one to two per day

Repetitions: eight to ten per exercise

Number of exercises: five in the beginner series; five in the intermediate series; five in the advanced series

Reevaluation of series M—N—O: Once the M series is easy, eliminate it and introduce the N series. Do the same progressing from the N series to the O series.

Table 4 Resistance Band Stabilization		
Series M Beginner	**Series N** Intermediate	**Series O** Advanced
Date:	Date:	Date:

In this table, just write the date of when you started the beginner series M, which you should do for up to six weeks before moving to the intermediate series N and another six weeks for the advanced.

Resistance Band M Series: Beginner

Exercise 1 – Hook-Lying Combination

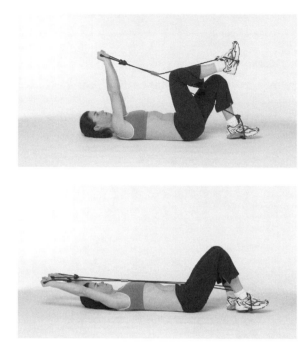

- Lying on your back, bend right hip and knee to 90 degrees, keeping your left foot on the floor, knee bent. Place the rubberband handles over each foot and in hands with the rubberband ropes passing over torso. Lift arms straight to 90 degrees over chest. Find neutral position. Do an abdominal set.

- Slowly lower your right leg to the floor, keeping knee bent to 90 degrees. Simultaneously lower both arms overhead, keeping elbows straight. Hold for five seconds. Slowly return to starting position.

- Do half of the repetitions on one side; change legs and complete the remainder of the repetitions.

Note: *Do not allow your back to arch.*

Exercise 2 – Half-Fold

- Lie on your back, knees bent, feet flat on floor. Place the rubberband handles over each foot. Have the rubberband ropes pass in between the legs and to the outside of the thigh. Place the opposite rubberband handles in each hand. Bring hands close to the ears by bending elbows. Find neutral position. Do an abdominal set.

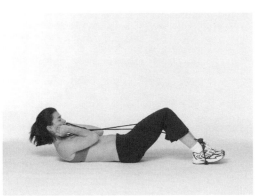

- Lift upper body (one vertebra at a time) into a crunch and reach toward knees. Shoulder blades should clear the floor. Keep your hands close to the ears at all times. Hold for five seconds. In the same manner, slowly return to starting position.

- Repeat.

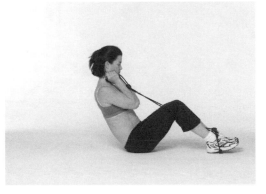

Note: *Always keep head looking forward at the knees, from the start to the finish position, to prevent tension at the neck.*

Exercise 3 – Bridging

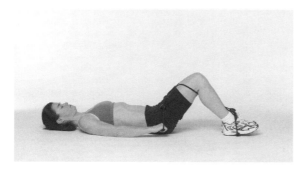

- Lie on your back, knees bent and feet flat on floor. Place the rubberband handles over each foot. Have the rubberband ropes pass in between the legs and crossed on the thighs. Place the other rubberband handles in each hand, with arms on each side of body. Find neutral position. Do an abdominal set.

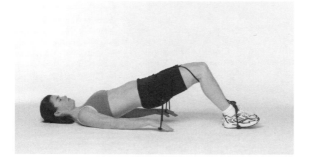

- Using buttock muscles, slowly raise pelvis from the floor, keeping trunk rigid and arms on the floor until pelvis is in line with knees and shoulders. Relax shoulders and neck. Hold for five seconds. Slowly return to starting position.

- Repeat.

Note: *Make sure not to do a pelvic tilt to raise hips or arch back to raise torso higher.*

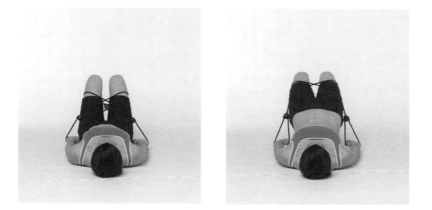

Exercise 4 – **Quadruped Lower Extremity Extension**

- Kneel on the floor, hands on the floor under shoulders, knees under hips. Keep spine straight and head aligned with spine. Place the rubberband handles over each foot. Have the rubberband ropes pass in between the legs and under torso on the floor. Place the other rubberband handles in each hand. Find neutral position. Do an abdominal set.

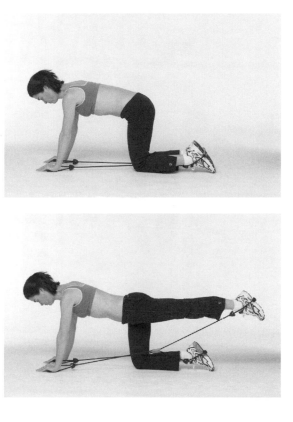

- Maintaining upper body alignment, slowly slide left leg along the floor until it is straight. Then using buttock muscles, lift left leg until it is parallel to the floor. Feel that you are stretching your leg toward the wall behind you instead of the ceiling above you. Keep pelvis and shoulders level. Hold for five seconds. Slowly return to starting position, keeping trunk rigid.

- Do half of the repetitions on one side, change legs and complete the remainder of the repetitions.

Note: *Do not allow your back to arch or to flex.*

Exercise 5 – Squats with Arm Curls

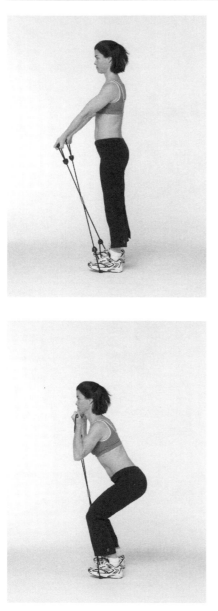

- Stand with chin at 90 degrees so that ears are in line with shoulders and shoulder blades are pulled down and inwards toward the spine. Place the rubberband handles over each foot and in hands with palms of hands facing the ceiling and arms at 45 degrees from body, keeping elbows straight. Have the rubberband ropes in front of you. Find neutral position. Do an abdominal set.

- Squat until hips are bent between 30 and 45 degrees. Simultaneously, curl arms toward chest, keeping wrists straight. Keep your body weight on your heels and maintain your abdominal set. Hold for five seconds. Slowly return to starting position.

- Repeat.

Note: *Do not allow your back to arch.*

Exercise 1 – Straight Leg Raise

- Lie on your back, left knee bent and left foot flat on floor, right hip bent to 45 degrees with knee straight so that right and left thighs are in line. Place the rubberband handles over each foot and hand with the rubberband ropes passing over torso. Lift arms straight to 90 degrees over chest. Find neutral position. Do an abdominal set.

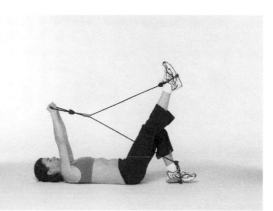

- While keeping your right knee straight, slowly lower your right leg until it is one inch above the floor. Simultaneously lower both arms overhead keeping elbows straight. Hold for five seconds. Slowly return to starting position.

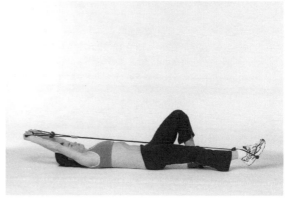

- Do half of the repetitions on one side; change legs and complete the remainder of the repetitions.

Note: *Do not allow your back to arch.*

Exercise 2 – The Fold

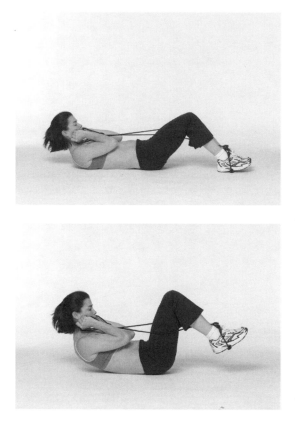

- Lie on your back, knees bent and feet flat on floor. Place the rubberband handles over each foot. Place the rubberband ropes in between the legs and to the outside of the thighs. Place the other rubberband handles in each hand. Bring hands close to the ears by bending elbows. Find neutral position. Do an abdominal set.

- Lift upper body (one vertebra at time) into a crunch until your shoulder blades are just off the floor. Keep your hands close to the ears at all times. Simultaneously curl hips off the floor by bringing knees toward elbows. Hold for five seconds. Slowly return to starting position.

- Repeat.

Note: *Always keep head looking forward at the knees, from the start to the finish position, to prevent tension at the neck.*

Exercise 3 – Bridging with Knee Extension

- Lie on your back, knees bent and feet flat on floor. Place the rubberband handles over each foot. Have the rubberband ropes pass in between the legs and crossed on the thighs. Place the other rubberband handles in each hand with arms on each side of the body. Find neutral position. Do an abdominal set.

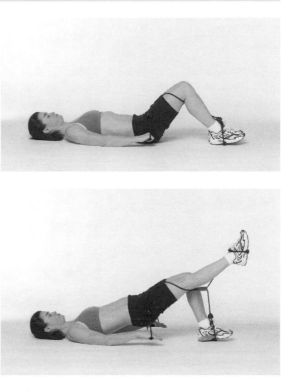

- Using buttock muscles, slowly raise pelvis from the floor, keeping trunk rigid until pelvis is in line with knees and shoulders. Slowly extend right leg from the knee without moving your pelvis, keeping trunk rigid. Both thighs should remain at the same level. Hold for five seconds. Slowly return to starting position.

- Do half of the repetitions on one side; change legs and complete the remainder of the repetitions.

Exercise 4 – Quadruped Opposite Upper/Lower Extremity Extension

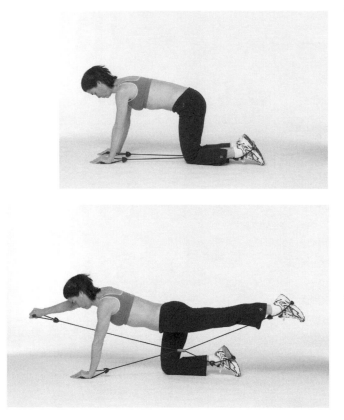

- Kneel on the floor, hands on the floor under shoulders, knees under hips. Keep spine straight and head aligned with spine. Place the rubberband handles over each foot. Have the rubberband ropes pass in between the legs and under torso on the floor. Place the other rubberband handles in each hand. Find neutral position. Do an abdominal set.

- Maintaining upper body alignment, slowly slide left leg along the floor until it is straight. Then using buttock muscles, lift left leg until it is parallel to the floor. Simultaneously, slowly slide right hand forward until arm is straight and lift right arm until it is parallel with the floor. Stretch in opposite directions, fingers and toes reaching for opposing walls of the room. Hold for five seconds. Slowly return to starting position, keeping trunk rigid.

- Do half of the repetitions on one side; change legs and complete the remainder of the repetitions.

Note: *Do not allow your back to arch or to flex.*

Exercise 5 – Plié with Front Raises

- Stand with chin at 90 degrees so that ears are in line with shoulders and shoulder blades are pulled down and inwards toward the spine. Turn your hips, legs, and feet outwards, at 45 degrees and shoulder-width apart. Place the rubberband handles over each foot and in hands with palms of hands facing the floor and arms at 45 degrees from body, keeping elbows straight. Have the rubberband ropes in front of you. Have your arms raised forward to 90 degrees, keeping elbows straight. Find a neutral position. Do an abdominal set.

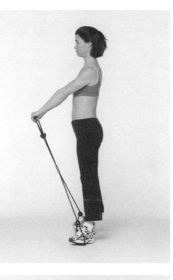

- Plié until upper thighs are between 30 and 45 degrees. Simultaneously, raise arms forward to 110 degrees. Keep your body weight back on your heels and maintain abdominal set. Hold for five seconds. Slowly return to starting position.

- Repeat.

Note: *Do not allow your back to arch.*

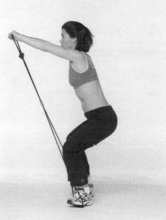

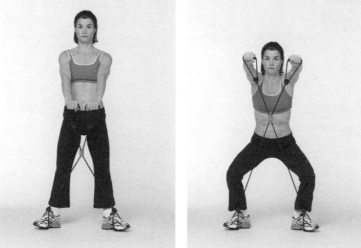

Resistance Band O Series: Advanced

Exercise 1 – Double Knee Lift

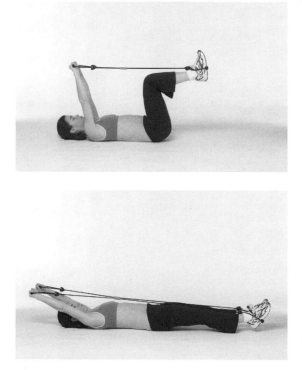

- Lie on your back with both hips and knees at 90-degree angles. Lift arms to 90 degrees over chest. Place the rubberband handles over each foot and hand with the rubberband handles passing over torso. Find neutral position. Do an abdominal set.

- Slowly straighten both legs from the hips and the knees until they are one inch above the floor. Simultaneously lower both arms overhead, keeping elbows straight. Hold for five seconds. Slowly return to starting position.

- Repeat.

Note: *Do not allow your back to arch.*

Exercise 2 – The V Position

- Sit on the floor. Bend hips to 90 degrees and knees to 45 degrees, feet flat on floor. Place the rubberband handles over each foot. Rest hands on floor, facing and behind buttocks, with elbows bent to 30 degrees, placing the other rubberband handles in each hand. Have the rubberband ropes passing in between the legs and on each side of the hips. Find neutral position. Do an abdominal set.

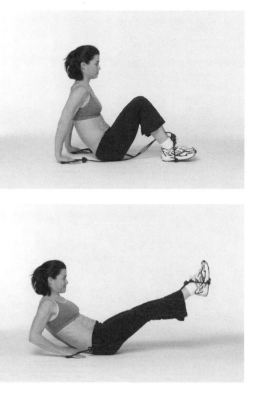

- Slowly extend your knees so that your legs are straight. Simultaneously bend elbows so that your upper body is at 45 degrees from the floor, keeping upper body straight. Hold for five seconds. Slowly return to starting position.

- Repeat.

Note: *Try to use stomach muscles instead of arms to hold upper body in position. And always keep head looking forward at the knees, from the start to the finish position, to prevent tension at the neck.*

Exercise 3 – Bridging with Straight Leg Raise

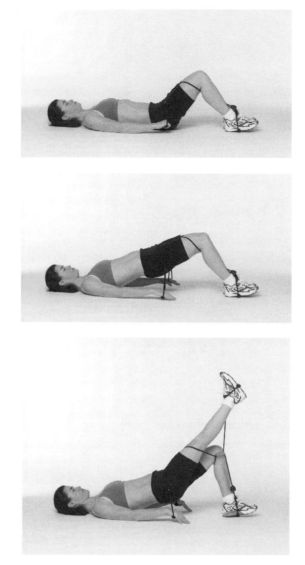

- Lie on your back, knees bent, feet flat on floor. Place the rubberband handles over each foot. Have the rubberband ropes pass in between the legs and crossed on the thighs. Place the other rubberband handles in each hand with arms on each side of the body. Find neutral position. Do an abdominal set.

- Using buttock muscles, slowly raise pelvis from the floor, keeping trunk rigid until pelvis is in line with knees and shoulders. Slowly extend the right leg from the knee like a hinge until leg is straight, keeping thighs in line. Flex right hip to your maximum hamstring flexibility (keeping knee straight, bring leg as far as possible toward head) without moving your pelvis and while keeping trunk rigid. Hold for five seconds. Slowly return to starting position.

- Do half of the repetitions on one side; change legs and complete the remainder of the repetitions.

Exercise 4 – Push-Up/Unilateral Hip Extension

- Begin in push-up position. Hands directly beneath shoulders and legs together, standing on your toes. Your body should be like a plank. Keep neck long and head aligned with your spine. Place the rubberband handles over each foot. Have the rubberband ropes passing under torso on the floor, and place the other rubberband handles in each hand.

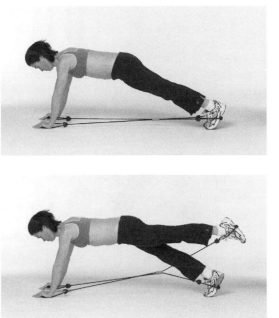

- Find neutral position. Do an abdominal set.

- Using your buttock muscles, raise left leg until it is parallel to the floor. Hold for five seconds. Slowly return to starting position, keeping trunk rigid.

- Do half of the repetitions on one side; change legs and complete the remainder of the repetitions.

Note: *Do not allow your back to arch. Keep body flat from your head to heels.*

Exercise 5 – Static Lunge with One Arm Front Raises

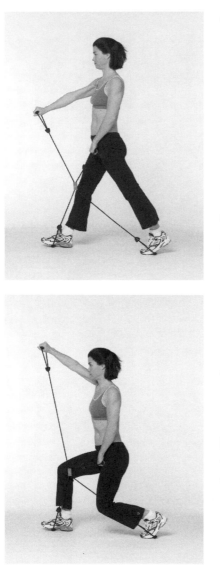

- Stand with right leg out in front of your body and the left leg behind on your tip-toes. Position chin at 90 degrees so that ears are in line with shoulders and shoulder blades are pulled down and inwards toward the spine. Place the rubberband handles over each foot and in each hand. Have right arm raised to 45 degrees in front of the body and left arm in front of left hip, keeping the rubberband ropes taut.

- Find neutral position. Do an abdominal set.

- Lower upper body by bending your left knee straight down to the floor. Do not allow the left knee to touch the floor. Simultaneously raise right arm to 110 degrees. Hold for five seconds. Slowly return to starting position, keeping trunk rigid.

- Do half of the repetitions on one side; change legs and complete the remainder of the repetitions.

Note: *Do not allow your front knee to bend more than 90 degrees or to extend in front of the front foot.*

References

Kapit, Wynn, and Lawrence M. Elson. 1977. *The Anatomy Coloring Book*. New York: Harper & Row.

Wharton, Jim, and Phil Wharton. 1996. *The Whartons' Stretch Book*. New York: Three Rivers Press.

Janique Farand-Taylor, PT, ACE, is a certified registered sports physiotherapist and certified personal trainer. She also practices craniosacral therapy and acupuncture. She owns a private practice in Toronto specializing in sports and orthopedic physical therapy. She is the official physiotherapist and personal trainer for the Ontario Freestyle Ski Team. She was a member of the Canadian Women's National Alpine Ski Team at the World Cup level from 1981 to 1985, and was selected for the Canadian Olympic Team at the 1984 Winter Olympiad in Sarajevo. She actively lectures; is a rehabilitative consultant to high school, college, and amateur sports teams; and is a freelance writer for Hockey Report Magazine.

Foreword writer **Ian Finkelstein, MD,** is a physician in private practive in Toronto, ON, Canada.

Some Other New Harbinger Titles

The Cyclothymia Workbook, Item 383X, $18.95

The Matrix Repatterning Program for Pain Relief, Item 3910, $18.95

Transforming Stress, Item 397X, $10.95

Eating Mindfully, Item 3503, $13.95

Living with RSDS, Item 3554 $16.95

The Ten Hidden Barriers to Weight Loss, Item 3244 $11.95

The Sjogren's Syndrome Survival Guide, Item 3562 $15.95

Stop Feeling Tired, Item 3139 $14.95

Responsible Drinking, Item 2949 $18.95

The Mitral Valve Prolapse/Dysautonomia Survival Guide, Item 3031 $14.95

Stop Worrying Abour Your Health, Item 285X $14.95

The Vulvodynia Survival Guide, Item 2914 $15.95

The Multifidus Back Pain Solution, Item 2787 $12.95

Move Your Body, Tone Your Mood, Item 2752 $17.95

The Chronic Illness Workbook, Item 2647 $16.95

Coping with Crohn's Disease, Item 2655 $15.95

The Woman's Book of Sleep, Item 2493 $14.95

The Trigger Point Therapy Workbook, Item 2507 $19.95

Fibromyalgia and Chronic Myofascial Pain Syndrome, second edition, Item 2388 $19.95

Kill the Craving, Item 237X $18.95

Rosacea, Item 2248 $13.95

Thinking Pregnant, Item 2302 $13.95

Shy Bladder Syndrome, Item 2272 $13.95

Help for Hairpullers, Item 2329 $13.95

Coping with Chronic Fatigue Syndrome, Item 0199 $13.95

The Stop Smoking Workbook, Item 0377 $17.95

Call **toll free, 1-800-748-6273,** or log on to our online bookstore at **www.newharbinger.com** to order. Have your Visa or Mastercard number ready. Or send a check for the titles you want to New Harbinger Publications, Inc., 5674 Shattuck Ave., Oakland, CA 94609. Include $4.50 for the first book and 75¢ for each additional book, to cover shipping and handling. (California residents please include appropriate sales tax.) Allow two to five weeks for delivery.

Prices subject to change without notice.